CHL̶O̶R̶E̶L̶L̶A̶: T̶H̶E̶ ̶P̶A̶T̶H̶W̶A̶Y̶ To Health, Vitality and Longevity

The whole food supplement that is nature's answer for today's most perplexing health problems.

Mark Drucker, M.D.

Donated by the family of
Jim Caldwell

Health and Happiness Publishing, Inc.

This publication is designed to provide accurate information with regard to the subject matter covered. It is never meant to be construed as medical advice or instruction, nor is it intended to replace medical diagnosis or treatment. Readers are strongly cautioned against self-treatment, and are urged to consult with appropriate health professionals on any matter relating to their health and wellbeing. Readers who fail to consult with appropriate health authorities assume risk of injury.

The author and publisher specifically disclaim any liability, loss, or adverse effects, personal or otherwise, that may be incurred by the indirect or direct use and application of any information contained in this book.

The information and opinion provided in the book are believed to be accurate and sound, based on the best judgment available to the author and publisher. The author and publisher are not responsible for errors or omissions.

First Edition
Copyright © 2002 by Health & Happiness Publishing

ISBN 0-96724681-4

Published by:
Health & Happiness Publishing
2435 E. North St #116
Greenville, SC 29615
http://www.health-books.com
Printed in the United States of America.

All of my knowledge, wisdom and inspiration comes from God, and this book is no exception. The true credit goes to our Heavenly Father and I am thankful for the opportunity to be of service. I would also like to thank my parents Jack and Lillian and my sister Myrna who gave me everything I needed to become someone who could help others on their road to health. Of course, I thank my wife Karin and my children Whitney and Brody who make it all worthwhile.

Biography

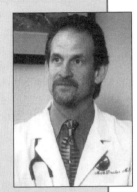

D r. Mark Drucker's medical career began 23 years ago. For the past 7 years, he has devoted his practice entirely to nutritional and natural medicine.

As co-founder and Medical Director for the Center for Advanced Medicine located in Encinitas, California, Dr. Drucker's practice is concentrated in a diverse range of specialties including; anti-aging medicine, natural hormone replacement, prolotherapy, chelation therapy, preventive medicine and detoxification.

Dr. Drucker is co-host of the popular syndicated radio talk show "Health Talk, A Second Opinion," which is focused exclusively on natural and nutritional therapies, as well as solving the "root cause of illness." As a frequent speaker on natural health topics, he conducts seminars and presentations in a variety of venues throughout the southwestern region of the United States.

Besides being a certified member of the American Academy of Anti-Aging Medicine--a society of physicians and scientists dedicated to enhancing the quality of life and extending human lifespans, Dr. Drucker is also a member of the American College for Advancement of Medicine. Additionally, he is a member of the American Academy of General Physicians, and a Diplomat Candidate of the American Board of Chelation Therapy.

Dr. Drucker received his bachelor's degree in biology from the University of Tennessee where he went on to receive his M.D. degree. His is a licensed physician in the states of California and Arizona.

Contents:

Preface

In all my years of searching for nutritional supplements for my patients, I've seen a lot of so-called "breakthroughs" come and go. New fads. Hot trends. Fabled discoveries. But when I heard about a natural whole food called chlorella, I knew I was onto something good. Here is a tiny water-grown plant with huge potential health benefits ranging from; healing ulcers and wounds, strengthening the immune system, promoting better digestion and elimination, protecting against occupational hazards such as industrial toxins and radiation exposure, reducing serum cholesterol and blood pressure, and assisting in gentle detoxification.

There are three main reasons why chlorella has helped many of my patients...even when drugs or typical treatments failed.

1. Chlorella is a potent stimulator of your body's natural defense system. The most powerful weapon we have against sickness and disease is the immune system. On a daily basis billions of immune cells battle against a constant barrage of enemies including: viruses, bacteria, parasites, and cancer — all threatening to attack from inside the body and out. In the Orient, traditional medical treatments often include natural substances derived from plants, mushrooms or microbial organisms such as algae and fungi. Known as "biological response modifiers," these substances improve the capacity of the body's immune system. Chlorella is well known in the Japanese scientific community as a biological response modifier. In fact, studies have consistently confirmed that chlorella can provide critical benefits for the health of individuals with suppressed immune systems caused by toxins, illness or side effects of conventional medical treatments.

2. Chlorella has been proven in numerous studies to have the ability to bind with, and remove chemicals and heavy metals, to relieve the body of its toxic burdens. Industrial toxins, heavy metals, carcinogenic chemicals, bacteria and a whole host of unwelcome visitors threaten our health daily. As I hold the tiny tablets of chlorella in my hand, the first thing that pops into my mind is how these "dark green wonders" can protect against a wide variety of toxic marauders lurking in the water we drink,

the food we eat, and the air we breathe. Toxic suppressors are, without controversy, the most destructive force in our world that robs us of our health. Although we can't completely avoid environmental toxins, clearly one of the most effective ways we can limit our exposure is by consistently taking a regular dose of this cleansing "superfood" with each meal.

3. Chlorella nourishes the body with valuable nutrients. Highly processed convenience foods have derailed our diets by substituting the "staff of life" found in whole grains, legumes, fruits and vegetables with complex carbohydrates such as processed flours, grains and sugars. As part of my practice, I stress to my patients the importance of eating plenty of fruits and vegetables, natural grains and other healthy foods. But with today's depleted soils, growing methods, processing and shipping methods, even "healthy" foods may be lacking some of the key vitamins, nutrients and minerals our bodies need. Chlorella is a concentrated source of unique, natural, non-synthetic nutrients. It can help provide critical nutritional support that certainly is lacking in the diets of most of us.

In my own practice, I've seen how chlorella has benefited many of my patients, especially those who take chlorella on a regular basis. I've had patients come in with extremely dangerous levels of chemical toxicity that was ruining their health and their lives. But chlorella, used along with other nutritional supplements, diet and natural treatments, has given many of these patients renewed health. Others have come to me suffering from a lifetime of chronic fatigue. Their body systems broken down. But chlorella has been one of the key elements in their recoveries.

One last point, chlorella is not a "magic pill" that will instantly cure whatever ails you. What chlorella does, however, is supply key nutrients that interact with the body systems in such a way as to enhance the body's ability to protect, balance and heal itself. While at the same time, chlorella removes the toxic suppressors that destroy health. These benefits are of critical importance for health, regardless of a person's condition. It might even be a "life saver" for individuals weakened by chronic illness. The benefits of chlorella are clear and simple. The mechanisms by which chlorella achieves these results are numerous and complex.

CHAPTER 1
Discovering The Green Wonder of the Orient

C hlorella is a single-celled fresh-water green algae packed with nutrients that can revolutionize your heath. Whether you suffer from life-threatening problems such as heart disease, arteriosclerosis, high blood pressure, diabetes and even cancer, or whether you endure chronic ailments like arthritis, sinus problems, joint pain, failing vision and fatigue, chlorella provides the perfect combination of nutrients that your body craves for healing itself.

Over 10 million people around the world use chlorella every day to supplement their diet. In Japan, chlorella is the best-selling health supplement. Classified as a food, chlorella has not been known to interfere with medications, and does not interact harmfully with other supplements. Instead, chlorella nourishes and revitalizes the cells of your body, providing you with more chlorophyll than any other plant, plus 18 amino acids, a variety of crucial minerals like iron, iodine, and zinc, essential fatty acids and beta-carotene.

Extensive scientific research proves that this microscopic green algae is indeed a phenomenal healer. According to the late Dr. Bernard Jensen, nutritional expert and author of *Chlorella: Gem of the Orient*, "chlorella is possibly the most thoroughly researched food of our times, with thousands of research papers, from many universities and medical schools." Numerous studies in Germany, the United States, Israel, England, China and Japan clinically document that chlorella can:

- boost the immune system, increasing your resistance to bacteria, viruses, chemicals and other foreign invaders.
- cleanse and remove toxins from your body, including pesticides and heavy metals.
- protect against cancer-causing agents and help to prevent cancer's recurrence.
- help repair damaged tissue and heal diabetic ulcers and wounds.
- protect the heart and reduce high blood pressure and cholesterol levels.
- promote brain wellness and fend off memory loss and Alzheimer's.

- regulate digestion and support proper bowel health.
- revitalize your energy level and stimulate your metabolism.
- reverse the aging process and promote longevity.

The Miracle of A Well-Nourished Body

Because chlorella performs so many therapeutic functions in the body, you may decide to take chlorella for one problem and then realize that it helps you with another. For instance, you may be interested in taking chlorella because you suffer from joint pain and then be thrilled to discover that not only is your pain diminished, but you are also sleeping better and losing weight.

Why? Because when you take chlorella, your body may become sufficiently nourished and cleansed for the first time in your life. We live in an age where food has been refined, processed, and stored in countless ways that destroy its nutrients. Plus, if we admit the truth, most of us don't eat a perfect diet anyway. The daily multi-vitamin that we take can't possibly furnish all the nutrients that we desperately need, and which our food is not completely supplying.

Furthermore, we live in a world bombarded by pollutants and chemicals that remain in our body, clogging our organs and compromising our immune system. These toxins drag down our energy level and make us vulnerable to every kind of disease.

But when you take chlorella, you'll experience two simultaneous miracles: a properly nourished body, and a system cleansed of toxins. The results will affect every aspect of your health, including some that may surprise you. You may find yourself walking with a spring in your step for the first time in years, radiant with new energy. And you may discover that with a detoxified, well-nourished body, your mood lightens and you feel happier, calmer and better able to handle the stress of everyday living.

Balancing Your System The Natural Way

One of the most intriguing aspects of chlorella is its unique ability to balance body functions, which is why some doctors have affectionately labeled it "the great normalizer." Dr. Randall E. Merchant, a clinical researcher from the Medical College of Virginia, Virginia Commonwealth University, says, "In testimonials that we've gathered over the years, we've found an interesting paradox. For people who take chlorella due to constipation - the constipation gets better. For people who take it for diarrhea - the diarrhea gets better. How can these two things happen? They

2

seem like opposites, but in both instances chlorella helps bring the body back into balance."

Here's another example of chlorella's amazing power to balance body functions—its effect on weight. Many people who take chlorella are delighted to discover that they effortlessly shed excess pounds, because chlorella stops their unhealthy cravings and stimulates their metabolism. However, if your body needs to hold onto its fat and resist losing weight, chlorella will help it do exactly that. A study of 971 sailors who endured a long, grueling tropical sea voyage showed that the 458 sailors who took chlorella maintained a healthy body weight, while those in the control group experienced serious weight loss. (It's also interesting to note that the sailors who took chlorella had 26.5% less colds.) [1]

2.5 Billion Years Old — And Still Going Strong

In recent years, chlorella has become increasingly popular in the United States. But chlorella is hardly a passing fad: it has been around for 2.5 billions years! In fact, chlorella is the oldest living organism on earth. It has survived in exactly this same form since the pre-Cambrian period, and is the first life form on earth to have a true nucleus.

Chlorella owes its unparalleled survival to two highly unusual characteristics. First, its cell wall is so tough that it is almost unbreakable. Second, it reproduces at an astonishing rate, rejuvenating into four new cells every seventeen to twenty hours.

Both of these qualities contribute to chlorella's unique healing powers. Its durable cell wall has the proven ability to bind with heavy metals, pesticides and toxins and carry them safely out of the body. And RNA and DNA, the driving forces behind chlorella's rapid reproduction, can powerfully stimulate growth, renewal and repair in humans. These nucleic acids, which can slow the aging process, are found in higher concentrations in chlorella than in any other known food.

One Cell, Many Nutrients

Only three to eight microns wide, chlorella is a whole food, meaning that you eat it in its entirety. Because each chlorella cell is a self-sufficient organism, all of its life forces are contained within it. Therefore, each cell provides you with a remarkably dense concentration of vital nutrients.

One of these nutrients is chlorophyll, which gives chlorella its deep green color. Known as the life blood of plants, chlorophyll is a superior blood builder, an extraordinary healer of wounds, and according to the late Dr. Bernard Jensen, "the greatest natural cleansing agent known to man." Chlorella has more chlorophyll per gram than any other plant. If you've been taking spirulina, wheatgrass or barleygrass, you'll be interested to know that chlorella contains five to ten times more chlorophyll.

As for protein, ounce for ounce, one gram of chlorella gives you almost twice as much as soybean and almost eight times as much as rice. That's because chlorella contains more than 50% protein, as well as 18 vitamins and minerals and a complete range of amino acids.

At the core of chlorella's healing powers is a unique chemical complex called Chlorella Growth Factor (CGF). All the elements within chlorella's nucleus — peptides, proteins, nucleic acids, polysaccharides and beta-glutens — combine to form CGF, which is a dynamo of therapeutic activity. CGF stimulates growth in children, repairs damaged tissue and protects your cells from toxins. Research shows that CGF is manufactured during the most intense periods of photosynthesis, incorporating within its structure the healing energy of sunlight.

The Evolution of Chlorella

The first laboratory culture of chlorella was developed in 1890 by a Dutch microbiologist named M.W. Beijerinck. In later decades, German scientists, intrigued by chlorella's high protein content, explored ways to turn it into food. After World War II, scientists from the United States took over the German research. A pilot study conducted at Stanford Research Institute proved decisively that chlorella could be grown and harvested in large quantities.

In 1951, the Rockefeller Foundation and the Japanese government co-sponsored a major research project on chlorella at the Kokugawa Biological Institute. Japan became the world pioneer in developing the technology to commercially produce chlorella. The rousing success of the Japanese project caught the attention of both the American and Russian space programs, who studied chlorella as an ideal food for long-term space travel and colonization.

But one huge obstacle remained before chlorella became the bestselling health supplement that it is today: it was largely indigestible. Chlorella's cell wall was so tough that it stayed intact in the body, making the nutrients inside the cell almost completely inaccessible. This problem was finally solved by a Japanese company, which after much research, developed a unique process that breaks down the cell wall, while preserving the nutritional value contained within.

Chlorella is grown in purified fresh mineral water pools outside in the sunshine. After the algae reach maturity, their walls are broken down and they are spray-dried and packaged into tablets. Each step of the process is conducted with the highest standards of sterility, and monitored constantly with state-of-the-art technology to maintain purity.

Green Gold for Every Member of the Family

The result is a supplement so brimming with health-giving properties that scientists around the world have nicknamed it "green gold," "the green wonder", and "gem of the Orient." Whatever you choose to call it, chlorella is clearly a superfood, a plant teeming with vital nutrients unmatched in their ability to restore and revitalize your overall well-being.

Every member of your family can enjoy chlorella. Whether you are a child needing nutritional support for growth, an adult worn down by never-ending stress or a senior citizen coping with the challenges of aging, chlorella will powerfully help and support you. It will boost your immune system and detoxify your body. It will fine-tune your metabolism, protect you from illness, regulate your digestion and turn back your aging process. It will increase your energy and elevate your mood. And most important of all, chlorella will help give you a longer life to enjoy the world around you and the people you love.

Someday in the future, space travelers may dine on chlorella. But today, we on earth have the opportunity to take chlorella and enjoy all the life-giving benefits of the greatest superfood of the 21st century.

CHAPTER 2
Chlorella, Nutritional Firepower for Your Immune System

Vicious Wars Inside Your Body

Every minute of the day, thousands of ferocious battles are raging inside your body. Hordes of microscopic foreign invaders are trying to penetrate your cells, while your body's hyperactive immune system struggles to fight them off. If the invaders win, the result could be an annoying cold that sidelines you for days. It could be a chronic illness that severely limits your enjoyment of life. Or, in extreme cases, it could be cancer or some other fatal disease.

According to *The Mayo Clinic Family Health Book*, "Agents that can invade your body live everywhere - in the air, on dust particles, food and plants, on and in animals and humans, in soil and water, and on virtually every other surface." Some of the most common ones are bacteria, viruses, fungi, yeast, parasites and environmental toxins. Your first layer of protection against these vicious invaders is your skin. But if they manage to sneak inside, the job of destroying them falls to your immune system.

That's why you want your immune system to be super-charged and ready to fight. You want your immune system primed to perform the complex task of instantly identifying dangerous intruders and formulating a specific response to destroy them. You want your white blood cells, the main soldiers of the immune system, able to race to the site of an infection, quickly surround the enemy and devour it until there's nothing left, or disarm it by neutralizing it and rendering it harmless.

But unfortunately, all too often, the immune system is not up to this never-ending challenge. A healthy immune system works at a frantic rate, constantly generating new cells. Many factors can dangerously slow down and suppress this process. Some of the most common ones are aging, exposure to chemical pollutants and inadequate nutrition.

When one or more of these factors weakens the immune system, it becomes sluggish and under-active. If your immune system is suppressed, it can not rally its troops to ward off the constant barrage of enemy intruders. The result is that you become more vulnerable to illness, from frequent colds that you cannot seem to get rid of, to cancerous tumors and other serious illnesses.

Chlorella Stimulates And Recharges Your Immune System

Fortunately, chlorella is a supreme booster of the immune system. Its nutrients are uniquely capable of addressing each of the factors that suppress the immune system, and stimulating recovery from their effects. A growing mountain of scientific data attests to chlorella's exceptional ability to empower the immune system, thereby preventing illness or dramatically lessening its impact.

Here are some clinical studies that show the range of chlorella's immune-boosting powers:

- As reported in *Cancer Immunology & Immunotherapy*, two groups of mice were injected with E. coli bacteria. The mice who were treated with chlorella extract experienced a "remarkable and significantly higher" accumulation of white blood cells to infection sites. In fact, the chlorella-treated mice had an incredible ten times the number of white blood cells than the controls! [2]

- Interferon is a protein produced in the body to fight viruses and other foreign agents. A 1990 study at the Department of Microbiology at Miyazaki Medical College studied the effect of chlorella on mice infected with an immune-suppressing virus, cytomegalovirus. Mice treated with chlorella showed a marked increased activity of interferon, as well as the natural killer activity of the body's spleen cells. This heightened immune activity saved the infected mice from death. [3] (figure 1)

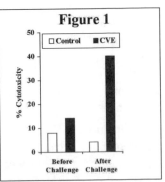

Figure 1

Effect of chlorella extract (CVE) on the NK (natural killer cell activity of spleen cells. Mice were treated with 10 mg of chlorella extract or a saline solution as a control, on days 3 and 1 before challenge with cytomegalovirus. The spleen cells of 5 mice per group were prepared from the treated mice at the time of challenge or on the 3rd day after challenge.

- *The International Journal of Immunopharmacology* reports that chlorella was given to mice infected with a virus similar to AIDS. The chlorella-treated mice had a "significantly higher" cell-mediated immune system response to the introduction of a bacterial infection, and a greater count of T-cells and B-cells, two of the most powerful warriors in the immune system. [4] (figure 2)

● Doctors at the Medical College of Virginia administered chlorella to patients with brain tumors. Patients who took chlorella achieved near-normal immune system blood cell counts and experienced fewer respiratory infections and flu-like illnesses. [5]

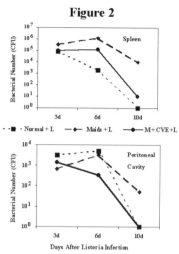

Figure 2

● Chemotherapy suppresses the white blood count, which is a significant problem in cancer treatment. In a study of mice treated with the chemotherapy drug 5-fluorouracil, those mice who were given a chlorella extract showed quicker recovery of white blood cells in bone marrow. Throughout the study, the chlorella group had a greater white blood cell count, and showed complete recovery of white blood cells 20% faster than the control group. [6]

Effect of oral administration of chlorella extract (CVE) on the growth of L. monocytogenes in the spleen and peritoneal cavity in mice infected with murine leukemia virus (MAIDS). Mice were infected with leukemia virus and challenged with L. monocytogenes on week 4 after leukemia virus infection. 2% chlorella extract-containing chows were given to infected mice on week 2 and continued until the experiment was over.

"I Haven't Had A Cold Since..."

The therapeutic results that scientists have found in the laboratory come as no surprise to chlorella's many devoted users. They know the difference that taking chlorella on a daily basis has made in their own lives.

Virginia Lindsteadt of Ukiah, California notes that chlorella prevents her sinus headaches and increases her energy. "My immune system has improved too. My overall health improved so much that I was able to work in Africa for six months in schools with children who have special needs. Some of the children were very ill, and during my time with them I never got ill. What a blessing!"

For those struggling to recharge their immune system and regain full health after an illness, Cecilia Weidmann of Miami, Florida offers some encouraging words. "Two and a half years ago I became very ill and had a near death experience. For a long time afterwards, I could not get my strength and stamina back. While discussing this with my doctor, he gave me literature on chlorella and told me to give it a try...In a couple of months, I felt like a new person. Recently, I was diagnosed with an immune deficiency…The cause is not known, but it can be very dangerous because I can pick up any type of infection and become seriously ill. My doctors are truly amazed that with my low globulin and white blood cell count, I remain in such good health…Other people with this condition that have higher globulin readings than mine become very ill. I feel chlorella has given my immune system the strength it needs to fight off infections."

4 Problems, 4 Solutions

To understand how chlorella revitalizes your immunity, let's take a closer look at its effect on four common problems of the immune system:

IMMUNE SYSTEM PROBLEM #1:
As you age, your immune system ages too.

Once you pass the vigor of adolescence, your immune system gradually becomes slower and less efficient. The thymus gland is the major culprit. It gradually shrinks, producing less thymosin, a hormone essential to your immune system's T-cells. But the problem extends to all your cells, which, as they grow older, become less adept at resisting infections.

THE SOLUTION:
Nourish your body with nucleic acids.

Chlorella has the highest concentration of nucleic acids of any food in the world. According to the late Dr. Benjamin S. Frank, author of *Dr. Frank's No Aging Diet*, a leading cause of aging is the breakdown of nucleic acids within the body. By nourishing your cells with RNA and DNA, the nucleic acids in chlorella, you help to halt the aging process that is diminishing your immune system.

Chlorella supplies your body with RNA, which is vital for producing the proteins that fight off infections, and DNA, which promotes healthy cell metabolism. Together, these health-giving nucleic acids work to delay the aging process and support the maximum capabilities of your immune system.

IMMUNE SYSTEM PROBLEM #2:
Inadequate nutrition.

According to an article published by The American Institute of Nutrition, "Malnutrition affects the structure and function of every tissue and physiologic system in the body, and the immune system is no exception. Protein-calorie malnutrition, or deficiencies of zinc, iron, selenium, pyridoxine and fatty acids, cause disruption in thymocyte-dependent cell-mediated immunity."

Unfortunately, the standard Western diet often falls short in delivering these vital nutrients. Even in affluent countries like the United States, surprising numbers of people suffer from protein deficiencies, because of bad eating habits and overly-processed food. Zinc, which is a key stimulant of the immune system, is also often lacking, particularly in older people. Along with pyridoxine (vitamin B-6), zinc enables your immune system to synthesize protein. Without healthy doses of all these nutrients, your immune system's troops are helpless when they face the enemy.

THE SOLUTION:
Chlorella delivers the nutritional firepower your immune system needs.

Chlorella's weight is 50% protein. That gives it a startling advantage in protein content over rice (7% protein by weight) and soybeans (39% by weight.). Taking chlorella on a daily basis helps to insure that your immune system constantly receives the protein it requires.

Additionally, chlorella contains zinc, pyridoxine (B-6), iron, and essential fatty acids. In the article quoted above, these are the very nutrients mentioned as necessary for a healthy immune system. By taking chlorella and supplying your body with adequate amounts of these important nutrients, you allow your immune system to operate at its peak. Your cellular weaponry will be stoked to seek out and destroy all dangerous intruders, be they bacteria, viruses, cancers, yeast, parasites, fungi or toxins.

IMMUNE SYSTEM PROBLEM #3:
Environmental Toxins.

We live in a world of constant chemical and environmental assaults. Day after day, your immune system is forced to cope with air pollution, artificial additives and residual pesticides in your food, waste-contaminated water, fumes from household cleaners, asbestos and much more. These toxins burrow into your system and refuse to budge. As they build-up, year after year, they seriously compromise your immune system. By breaking down your cellular defenses, these toxic invaders leave you exhausted and increasingly vulnerable to disease.

THE SOLUTION:
Chlorella cleanses toxins from the body and safely sweeps them out.

Unlike spirulina or other "green products," chlorella has sticky cell walls which bind themselves to toxins, wrap them up and escort them out of the body. This unique, absolutely priceless ability means that toxic intruders, which could cause cancer and other diseases, are permanently removed from your body. One of the most important results of this cleansing is that your immune system is freed from the destructive impact of these toxins and can operate at higher capacity.

In addition to its cell walls, chlorella has another powerful cleanser: chlorophyll, nature's most powerful detoxifying agent. Chlorella has the highest percentage of chlorophyll of any known plant, which is another reason chlorella is such an important ally of your immune system.

IMMUNE SYSTEM PROBLEM #4:
Attack by Free Radicals.

As part of its normal functioning, your body uses oxygen. The by-products of this process are short-lived molecules called "free radicals," which roam through your system, attacking cell membranes and genetic materials. Free radicals have been associated with cancer, heart disease, Alzheimer's and other serious diseases. Although they are created naturally in the body, they are also unleashed by sunlight, air pollution, smoke, alcohol and unsaturated fats.

The immune system is greatly weakened by contact with free radicals and can sustain heavy blows in its ability to defeat disease. The way to fight back is through antioxidants, which have the power to neutralize free radicals. Unfortunately, most people don't get enough antioxidants in their diet, a problem which increases as they age.

THE SOLUTION:
Chlorella is power-packed with antioxidants.

Antioxidants are well-known for their ability to fight free radicals. Chlorella contains a powerful arsenal of antioxidants. This makes chlorella an astonishingly potent warrior against free radicals.

Chlorella contains an impressive six times more beta-carotene than spinach, an antioxidant renowned for its cancer-fighting abilities. Your body converts beta-carotene to vitamin A and uses it to fortify cell membranes, so they can better resist enemy penetration.

By nourishing your body with chlorella's antioxidants, you help fend off the devastating damage of free radicals on your immune system and protect yourself from a host of serious diseases.

Give Yourself The Gift Of A Healthy Immune System

If you are concerned about your health, one of your top priorities must be taking care of your immune system. As the saying goes, "a strong defense is the best offense." By insuring that your immune system's soldiers are battle-ready and armed to the hilt, you prevent disease from ever gaining a foothold in your cells. While others around you come down with every passing bug, you can still perform at your peak ability. And, year after year, you remain tumor-free and resistant to serious chronic illnesses.

That's why chlorella is such a valuable part of your self-care regimen. By taking chlorella on a regular basis, you can:

- increase the efficiency of your cell metabolism.
- support the production of interferon, a powerful natural anti-viral agent.
- elevate your white blood count.
- destroy cancer-bearing agents.
- resist colds, viruses and flus.
- lessen the severity of an illness, and recover more quickly from it.

These unrivaled therapeutic powers have inspired Dr. Randall E. Merchant, head of Neurosurgery, to say, "The research I have been and continue conducting at the Medical College of Virginia has convinced me that chlorella is clearly the most powerful natural food you can take daily to support and enhance your immune system function."

CHAPTER 3

Removing Industrial Toxins from Your System — The Natural Way!

O nce upon a time, our air was fresh and our water was clean. Most people lived and worked on farms where they ate wholesome food which they grew themselves. Human exposure to toxic chemicals was minimal.

Today our air is clogged with dangerous pollutants from car emissions and industrial by-products. Our water is contaminated with sewage and run-off from chemical factories. And our food is loaded with artificial additives and pesticides.

Everywhere we go, toxic chemicals assail us, even in places we least expect them: the carpets we walk on, the cologne we splash on our face, the pots we cook in and the dental fillings in our mouth.

The sad truth is that modern life is an unsupervised experiment in toxic bombardment. No one knows what the end result will be, but the enormous number of people suffering from cancer, respiratory problems, chronic fatigue and other ailments indicates that the price of modernity may be serious disease.

Numbers Tell the Dirty Truth

Take a look at some of these staggering statistics:

- In 1989 alone, the amount of chemical pollutants released into the environment was 5,705,670,380 pounds.

- 64,000 people die every year in urban America from lung or heart problems caused by air pollution. (Los Angeles Times, May 9, 1996)

- Since 1940, we have increased the number of synthetic chemicals in the environment by 380 times.

- The average person today has 1000 times more lead in their body than people living 500 years ago. (Claire Patterson, Ph.D., California Institute of Technology)

- 25 billion pounds of synthetic chemicals are released into the market every year.

By sending huge quantities of toxins into the environment, we invite a public health disaster. Heavy metals, like mercury, lead and aluminum, can linger in your body for decades, creating havoc with your physical well-being. In the words of Dr. Michael E. Rosenbaum, toxic chemicals become a "hazardous dump site in need of major clean up - right in your very own body!"

What exactly do toxins do? Increasing evidence links heavy metals and environmental pollutants to Alzheimer's, heart disease, cancer, neurological disorders and other serious ailments. Toxins are associated with the creation of free radicals. Toxins suppress your immune system, rob your energy and increase your chances for malignant tumors and other diseases. And decade after decade, they can remain in your cells, creating ever-more serious trouble.

The Natural Way To Detoxify Your Body of Toxins

The difficulty of dislodging toxins once they have settled into your body is one reason why so many scientists are excited about chlorella. This "green wonder" possesses a unique ability to bind to toxins and safely evict them from the body. Dr. David Steenblock, author of *Chlorella: Natural Medicinal Algae*, writes "Chlorella has been shown to remove toxic insecticides and pesticides. It has been shown to remove P.C.B. and DDT, cadmium, lead and other heavy metals. In today's world of constant chemical exposure, chlorella's ability to detoxify the body of dangerous environmental pollutants is of great significance."

Chlorella owes its remarkable detoxifying powers to two elements: its cell wall and its high chlorophyll content. The cell wall is an extremely adhesive, almost unbreakable membrane that sticks to toxins, wraps them up and permanently removes them from the body. No other cell wall, including that of spirulina, is known to possess these detoxifying powers. Chlorella also contains the highest chlorophyll content of any plant in the world. A supremely potent cleansing agent, chlorophyll helps give chlorella its unmatched detoxifying abilities.

Health Destroyers and Health Restorers

Let's look at some common toxic culprits, and some exciting studies of chlorella's ability to detoxify them from your body:

Cadmium:

A heavy metal that attacks the immune system. By weakening your ability to fend off disease, cadmium encourages the growth of bacteria, viruses, fungi and parasites. According to the United States Environmental Protection Agency, short-term exposure to cadmium may result in nausea, vomiting, diarrhea, muscle cramps, salivation, sensory disturbances, liver injury, convulsions, shock and renal failure. People with long-term cadmium build-up may experience kidney, liver, bone and blood damage.

Exposure: Cigarette smoke is a leading cause of cadmium exposure, but it's not the only one. Researchers at the Memorial University of Newfoundland, Saint Johns in Canada, state that cadmium "is virtually absent from tissues at birth, but is gradually accumulated, so that in a lifetime an average person living in an industrial society stores a substantial amount of cadmium in his body." Cadmium can make its way into drinking water from plumbing, industrial waste and leaching of landfills. Seafood is another source, as is the backing of carpets.

Cadmium is used in metal plating, and in the manufacturing of paints, plastic batteries, and many other products. People who work in these fields are in greater danger of cadmium build-up because of their increased exposure.

Chlorella Studies: A Japanese study by Hagino et al. studied the effects of chlorella on patients suffering from cadmium poisoning. Doctors gave patients eight grams of chlorella daily. After 12 days, cadmium in the excretions of the patients increased three times over the baseline. After 24 days of chlorella, the cadmium in the urine had increased seven times greater than baseline and patients reported significant reduction of pain. The conclusion reached by Hagino et al. is that chlorella acted as a detoxifying agent to remove cadmium via the urine. [7]

Dr. David Steenblock reports "chlorella binds strongly to cadmium and will not give it up to the body." In 1978, researchers proved this point in an experiment in which rats were given chlorella bound with cadmium. A control group was given only cadmium. The control group showed retardation of growth and cadmium in the blood. The group given chlorella showed no growth retardation and no cadmium in the blood, proving that chlorella allowed the cadmium to pass through the body with no effect. [8]

Research shows that zinc prevents "cadmium-induced suppression of the immune system." [9] Chlorella is a natural source of zinc.

Mercury:

A poisonous liquid metal that accumulates in the body for years. According to the Environmental Protection Agency, mercury can cause cancer and damage to the brain, kidneys, stomach, intestine and lungs.

Mercury permanently harms unborn children and increases blood pressure and heart rate. It is also associated with chronic fatigue syndrome, neurological damage, depression and anxiety.

Exposure: From 1987 to 1993, nearly 68,000 pounds of mercury were released into land and water. Mercury accumulates in fish, and does not dissipate even when cooked. The Food and Drug Administration warns pregnant women against eating shark, swordfish, king mackerel and tilefish, because their high mercury content can damage a fetus's brain.

Another source of mercury contamination is dental fillings. Almost all of the fillings in the United States are "silver" amalgams which contain mercury. It's a matter of controversy as to how safe these fillings are, but evidence increasingly suggests that they can contaminate the body. The governments of Sweden and Denmark have recommended against using fillings with mercury and Germany has cautioned against its use in pregnant women.

Chlorella Studies: A Canadian study reports on 60 patients suffering from various painful symptoms attributed to mercury poisoning. These patients were treated with chlorella to detoxify them, and then had their dental amalgam fillings replaced. Seventy-eight percent reported that they were either satisfied or very satisfied with the results of treatment. [10]

In *Chlorella Natural Medicinal Algae*, Dr. Steenblock notes a study in which "brewer's yeast culture was poisoned and killed by the addition of P.C.B., mercury, copper and cadmium. When chlorella extract was added to these toxic substances, the brewer's yeast remained alive!"

The Dental Amalgam Mercury Syndrome newsletter recommends chlorella as a natural detoxifying agent for people with accumulated mercury levels. [11]

A clinical study proved that chlorella successfully removes mercury from the bowels and cells. An additional study proved chlorella acts as an ion exchange resin in the stomach, thereby removing mercury from blood. [12]

Other studies have proven chlorella's ability to detoxify such heavy metals as uranium and lead. Lead is implicated as a risk factor in Alzheimer's and affects brain cells and the nervous system. Even if you avoid eating or drinking from ceramic dinnerware made with lead glazes, you still run the risk of toxic exposure. Household pipes often corrode, filling your tap water with unacceptable lead levels. And mining and smelting operations can pollute your local water sources. In a recent six year period, 144 million pounds of lead compounds were released into land and water.

One of the most worrisome aspects of lead exposure is its effect on children. Delays in physical and mental development in babies and young children are common, and some children suffer permanently reduced intelligence, hearing and attention span.

Welcome News For A Toxic World

That's why, in an evermore polluted world, chlorella offers a green beacon of hope. The well-documented ability of chlorella's cell walls to bind to a toxin, wrap it up, and safely remove it from your body, coupled with the cleansing power of its high chlorophyll content, gives you a simple, natural way to reduce the long-term build-up of heavy metals and other chemical pollutants in your system. Left unchecked, these toxins could gradually destroy your health, inviting Alzheimer's, cancer, kidney disease, chronic fatigue and other major problems to rob you of the chance to enjoy a long, vital life.

Here's a list of people who should be particularly concerned about toxic build-up in their bodies. Take a look and see if you or someone you love is on it.

- People whose job exposes them to chemicals through manufacturing, mining, smelting or other processes.
- People in areas of heavy air pollution.
- People in manufacturing regions where toxins could leak into the water supply.
- People with dental fillings containing mercury.
- Children who may be exposed to lead. (The tap water of 30 million Americans contains potentially dangerous levels of lead.)
- Pregnant women and women of child-bearing years who can pass toxins onto their unborn baby.
- People who eat large quantities of fish.
- People whose houses have old plumbing that may corrode and pass on contaminants.

If you are concerned about the possibility of long-term exposure to toxins, chlorella can help ease your mind. By taking chlorella on a daily basis and continually sweeping toxins from your body, you can protect your health and very possibly increase your life span. In an environment booby-trapped with dangerous chemicals, you can breathe more freely and deeply, knowing that the cleansing magic of chlorella is working for you.

CHAPTER 4

You Are What You Eat: Protecting Against Carcinogens and Chemicals in Your Food

A golden peach that gushes rivers of sweet juice into your mouth. A tangy spinach salad festooned with tender-green slices of avocado. A thick burger served sizzling hot off the grill. How delicious all these foods are and how healthy-sounding. But along with their scrumptious flavor, they also could be serving up a hidden army of cancer-causing chemicals.

Consider some alarming facts: every year, 2 billion pounds of pesticides are sprayed on American crops. Inevitably, significant amounts wind up in the food we eat. According to *The New York Times,* "pesticide residues are omnipresent in the American food supply: the Federal Drug Administration finds them in 30 to 40 percent of the food it samples. Many of them are known carcinogens, neurotoxins and endocrine disrupters - dangerous at some level of exposure. The government has established acceptable levels for these residues in crops, though whether that means they're safe to consume is debatable, in setting these tolerances the government has historically weighed the risk to our health against the benefit — to agriculture that is. The tolerances also haven't taken into account that children's narrow diets make them especially susceptible, or that the complex mixture of chemicals to which we're exposed heighten the dangers."

A recent survey of pesticide residues by the Department of Agriculture painted a surprising picture: contrary to the popular belief that domestic produce is safer than imported produce, the government discovered 11 of the 12 most contaminated fruits and vegetables were grown in the United States. Apples, on average, contained 4 pesticides, but some had 10. And one single sample of spinach contained a whopping 14 different pesticides![13]

"We Still Find Background Levels of DDT"

Among the pesticides turning up in the government survey was

Dieldrin, which was banned more than 25 years ago. Like many pesticides ruled illegal after their cancer-causing properties were found, Dieldrin lingers in the soil for decades. *The New York Times* quotes Harry Leichtwas, a senior research analytical chemist at General Mills. Not only does Mr. Leichtwas test the 400 pesticides currently approved by the EPA, but also the dozens of others that have been banned over the years as their dangers became evident. "Decades later, many of these toxins remain in the soil and continue to show up in our food. We still find background levels of DDT and chlordane," he explained.

Pesticides are not the only undesirable chemicals in our food. More than 2,800 food additives are currently listed by the Food and Drug Administration. The result: the average American eats or drinks almost 10 pounds of them every year. How do all these food additives collectively interact? No one can begin to say.

This unending chemical saturation leaves those of us concerned about our health in a quandary. We need to eat, and we want to eat. In fact, good food is one of life's most unbeatable pleasures. But even if we decide to do our health a favor and emphasize fruits and vegetables in our diet, we could wind up eating large quantities of foods that are dangerously riddled with poisons.

1 in 4 Deaths In America Is From Cancer

The end result is that many of us worry about cancer. Maybe we had the misfortune of experiencing cancer ourselves. Or perhaps a friend, a neighbor, a colleague or even someone we love has suffered through the horror of cancer diagnosis and treatment. Sometimes it seems that cancer is everywhere, and with good reason. Cancer is the second leading cause of death in the United States, exceeded only by heart disease. Every day, 1,500 Americans die of cancer, a total of more than five million lives lost since 1990.

With carcinogens lurking in our breakfast, lunch and dinner, what can we do to protect ourselves? What are the steps we can take to reduce our risk and fortify our systems against the onslaught of cancer-causing agents in our food and drink?

Nature's Green Gift At The Forefront of Cancer Research

One of the simplest, most effective steps you can take is to add chlorella to your daily routine. This nutrient-packed algae is at the forefront of cancer research and the subject of a growing mountain of scientific literature that confirms its cancer-fighting prowess. Chlorella protects you from cancer in a number of important ways. Its cell wall binds to pesticides and insecticides that may be lodged in your body, and safely sweeps them out. Its chlorophyll content effectively detoxifies a host of cancer-causing toxins. And its combination of nutrients strongly stimulates your immune system, enabling it to destroy cancer-causing cells and resist tumor growth.

The proof is in the laboratory, where a stream of exciting data attests to chlorella's cancer-beating gifts. In a study published in *Drug and Chemical Toxicology*, scientists led by Dr. Pore of West Virginia University, administered chlorella to a group of rats injected with chlordecone, a harmful insecticide. The rats with chlorella eliminated chlordecone from their system at more than twice the rate of the control group. The chlorella passed through the gastrointestinal tract unharmed, interrupted the recirculation of the insecticide, and eliminated the bound chlordecone with the feces. [14] This study supports research at the Fukuoka Institute for Health and Environmental Sciences in Japan, where scientists successfully used chlorophyll to speed the elimination of dioxin from rats, a toxin often found in meat. [15]

Of course, chlorella doesn't just help rats. It helps people too. Dr. Ueda, of the Institute for Environmental Pollution Research in Japan, gave chlorella to 30 patients suffering from exposure to the pesticide P.C.B. (polychlorobiphenyl). Over a one year period, almost all patients experienced higher energy levels, achieved better digestion and normal bowel movements. [16]

...And A Side of Chlorella, Please

If you are like most Americans, you love to eat meat. You enjoy chomping into a towering roast beef sandwich or gobbling down a thick juicy steak. Unfortunately, there's sad news for meat lovers. By eating your favorite foods, you could be promoting cancer of your colon and stomach. When meat is cooked at high temperatures, by broiling, frying or barbecuing, cancer-causing chemicals called heterocyclic amines (HCAs) are formed. In fact, those delicious brown bits on your steak and the charcoal lines on your hot dogs are laden with HCAs.

Now for the good news. Chlorophyll is a remarkably effective fighter of HCAs and other toxins found in meat. In a wealth of studies, chlorophyll inhibited the uptake of HCAs in the large and small intestines and the liver, and at its highest dose, completely prevented any uptake. [17]

In order to be most effective, chlorophyll should be taken at the same time as the HCAs. [18] That's a good motive to take chlorella as a side dish with your steak, because chlorella contains more chlorophyll than any organism in the world.

Researchers at Oregon State University and the University of Hawaii have identified other carcinogens that chlorophyll can successfully vanquish. Among them aflatoxin B1. *Cancer Research Journal* of January 1995 reports that these findings have "important implications in intervention and dietary management of human cancer risks." [19] And a recent issue of *Carcinogenesis* notes that chlorophyll inhibits formation of mutation by forming a chemical bonding with cancer-causing substances in meat, and suppressing a cancer-promoting enzyme. [20]

Reducing the Incidence of Tumors

The best way to prevent cancer is to cleanse toxins from your system, and short-circuit tumors before they get started. But if tumors are already secretly forming inside your body, chlorella can provide essential support so that the immune system can more effectively combat the tumor.

In a study sponsored by The American Cancer Society, researchers at Yale and Seoul, Korea investigated chlorophyllin's effect against certain carcinogens. All the mice in the control group formed skin tumors. But the mice which had been pretreated with chlorophyllin had 42% fewer tumors and papillomas. [21]

In a Japanese study, tumor mass disappeared in 50% of mice receiving a chlorella extract. In the control group, tumors progressed until all the mice died. [22] Another study found a 66-100% inhibition in the spread of tumors in mice given a chlorella extract 10 days before they were rechallenged with identical tumors cells. The mice which received the most concentrated doses of one of the most potent glycoproteins found in chlorella extract were completely free of tumors. [23]

How does chlorella inhibit tumor growth or make them disappear? The answer seems to lie in its vigorous stimulation of the immune system. The scientists who conducted the Japanese study on tumor mass in mice reported that the chlorella extract worked by enhancing the immune system's T-cell activity, and mobilizing those cells to infiltrate tumor sites. [22,23]

These cancer-fighting properties can give you mighty protection against the daily barrage of chemicals in your food and drink. With a revved-up immune system, your body can activate the necessary cells to engulf and destroy carcinogens and stop tumors in their tracks.

Chlorella to The Rescue: Bacteria, Watch Out!

Of course, toxic chemicals aren't the only danger that can lurk in your food. Deadly bacteria can hide there, too. In 1999, 35 million pounds of ready-to-eat meats were recalled, including batches of brand name hot dogs, deli meats, smoked fish and chicken, after widespread contamination with Listeria monocytogene was discovered.

Listeria is a food-borne bacteria that can be fatal, especially to people with weak immune systems, such as the elderly, pregnant women and babies. Four-hundred twenty-five people died of Listeria in 1998. Although it is killed by cooking and pasteurization, Listeria can contaminate ready-to-eat meats after they are processed. Your salad might also be a source of this frightening bacteria, because manure from infected animals can spread it into the soil that your carrots grow in.

Fortunately, chlorella boosts your immune system so that it can better fight off Listeria. A control group of mice was not given chlorella and infected with Listeria. All the mice died. But an infected group given a chlorella extract had a 20 to 55% survival rate, depending on the dose. The survival of the mice was attributed to increased activity of their immune system's natural killer cells. [24] (figure 3)

Chlorella also worked wonders against another fatal bacteria, E. coli. When mice with suppressed immune systems were given chlorella extract, they succeeded in eliminating lethal doses of E. coli. But the mice who did not receive the chlorella extract died within 24 hours. [2]

Figure 3

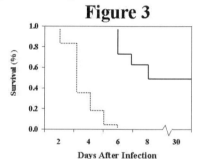

Days After Infection

Effect of oral administration of chlorella extract (500mg/Kg/day) on survival ratio of mice infected with lethal dose of L. monocytogenes. Treated and infected group (—); infected group (...).

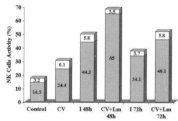

Effect of oral administration of chlorella (CV) extract (500mg/Kg/day) on the NK (natural killer) cells activity of L. monocytogenes infected mice, observed at 48 hours and 72 hours after infection.

A Banquet of Food Served With Peace of Mind

Consider a tempting dinner spread before you. That healthy-looking salad could bear residues of the multiple pesticides with which it was sprayed. Your steamed string beans may have been grown in soil that is still contaminated by DDT or other pesticides banned decades ago. Your steak can contain dioxin in its fats and cancer-causing HCAs. And your salad dressing, dinner roll, instant rice and chocolate pudding are all laced with dozens of food additives that combine in unknown ways. To top it all off, dangerous bacteria could lurk anywhere. What on earth can you do?

Here's your green insurance policy: take chlorella with your meal. Its nutrients go to work on your behalf, evicting cancer-causing toxins from your system before they burrow in. They stimulate your immune system, helping it to infiltrate and destroy growing tumors. And they provide you with powerful ammunition against disease-causing bacteria.

So serve up peace of mind along with your broccoli. Add a healthy serving of chlorella to your menu.

CHAPTER 5

Nourishing Every Cell: Chlorella, The Ultimate Superfood

Taking a trip to your local health supplement store can be a bewildering experience. You stand in front of endless rows of shelves, gazing from one bottle to another. Which vitamins are you supposed to take for your condition? Which minerals? If you are already taking a vitamin, should you add another? As for herbs and other supplements, which ones interfere with your medication? What are the best brands? How can you tell the right dosage?

Finally you shrug and walk away. Who has the patience — or the money — to deal with all these choices? Besides, you already find it a challenge keeping track of your various supplements and medications.

If you have ever had a similar experience, you will be relieved to know that in a world of complicated choices, there does exist one perfect food: chlorella. Combining a wealth of vitamins, minerals, proteins, amino acids and other vital nutrients into a simple hard-working whole food, chlorella powerfully delivers the wide-range of nutrition your body needs.

And, most importantly, chlorella is classified as a food, meaning that it will not interfere with any medication you may be taking. You can add chlorella to your diet, as confidently as you would spinach or broccoli. Its targeted nutrition will go to work for your body, healing and protecting, without ever compromising the efficiency of your prescription medicine. However, it is always a good idea to consult your physician about the addition of this vital whole food to your daily regimen.

Whole, Pure And Natural: The Perfect Food

According to the late Dr. Bernard Jensen, chlorella is "a whole food because each cell is a complete plant, with all of its life attributes intact. It's a pure food, uncontaminated by chemicals or pesticides. It's a natural food, with nothing added and nothing taken away."

Let's take a look at some of chlorella's key nutrients and their formidable healing powers:

Chlorella Growth Factor (CGF): Only one organism in the world contains this miraculous rejuvenator: chlorella. In *Chlorella: Gem of the Orient*, Dr. Jensen wrote "If I had to pick out the most valuable features of chlorella in preventing disease and lifting the general health level, I would give CGF and the nucleic acids in it the most credit, because they lift the energy level of the body *as a whole* and because they repair and renew *all* organs, glands and tissues of the body." Derived from the nucleus of the chlorella cell, CGF is the engine that drives chlorella's rapid regeneration, allowing it to reproduce every 20 hours. Studies show that CGF not only maintains and repairs cells, it also supports the immune system, stimulates new cell growth and increases energy levels. Created during the most intense periods of photosynthesis, CGF gives chlorella the highest concentration of nucleic factors (up to 13% RNA and DNA) of any known food.

Chlorophyll: Chlorella's deep green color comes from its high density of chlorophyll, the health-giving nutrient known as the "life-blood" of plants. Long renowned for its healing powers, chlorophyll is the most powerful natural detoxifying agent in the world, capable of sweeping heavy metals and toxins out of the body. Chlorophyll is almost identical in structure to hemoglobin (red blood cells), and is a remarkably effective agent for tissue growth and repair. It also is associated with healthy respiration, efficient digestion, and the reduction of body odors. Chlorella contains more chlorophyll per gram than any other plant.

Protein: Chlorella contains 50 to 60% protein, giving it twice as much protein per gram as steak! Protein is essential to the human metabolism,

The Chlorella Growth Factor (CGF)	Chlorophyll	Protein
That helps you... • Maintain and repair cells • Increase energy levels • Stimulate growth of new cells • Support immune function	*That helps you...* • Rid your body of damaging toxins and free radicals • Avoid the appearance of premature aging • Cleanse heavy metals and toxins from the body • Support respiratory function • Promote healthy digestion • Improve feelings of well-being • Reduce body odors	*That helps you...* • Repair and rebuild damaged tissues • Boost your energy naturally • Curb food cravings
Amino Acids		**Polysaccharides (beta glucan)**
That helps you... • Boost your body's natural defense system • Support and maintain healthy immune function • Put yourself at less risk for infection and virus-related illnesses	**Beta-Carotene Antioxidant** *That helps you...* • Fight off free radical damage • Build-up immune system • Combat the effects of free radical damage • Protect the skin • Promote proper circulation	*That helps you...* • Deter free radicals • Support your body in its efforts to fight infection • Increase immune function
		Unique Fiber *That helps you...* • Support and maintain healthy digestion

and even in affluent Western countries, is often lacking in many people's diets. Without protein, cells can not grow or repair themselves. Chlorella has twice as much protein as soybeans and seven times as much as rice.

Amino Acids: Amino acids are the building blocks for cell repair and maintenance. Chlorella contains all 8 essential amino acids, including lysine, which is frequently lacking in our high wheat diets, and arginine, which boosts the immune system's production of disease-fighting T-cells. According to Dr. Michael E. Rosenbaum, chlorella "is one of the very few foods, from a non-meat based source, that offers the vegan or vegetarian the complete spectrum of amino acids needed to support optimal health."

Beta-Carotene Antioxidant: Free radicals are short-lived molecules that roam through your body, attacking your cells and unleashing serious diseases. The best way to fight free radicals is with antioxidants, and chlorella is a superb source of these. Containing a variety of antioxidant carotenes, chlorella is particularly rich in beta-carotene, supplying six times more of this cancer-fighting agent than spinach. Carotenes are also known to be essential nutrients for supporting brain wellness and the immune system.

Vitamins: Chlorella contains an impressive array of natural vitamins, including vitamin A, a major booster of the immune system. Ounce for ounce, it contains more B-12 than beef liver, as well as vitamins B-1, B-2, B-6, E, niacin and the powerful heart helper, pantothenic acid.

Minerals: Zinc is crucial to your health. Dr. Michael E. Rosenbaum writes that zinc "is the most important nutrient for your immunity. It is a potent immunostimulant and a co-factor in over 80 enzyme reactions in your body." In addition to having ample amounts of zinc, chlorella also contains iron, magnesium, iodine and phosphorus.

Meet the Superfood of the 21st Century

Because chlorella contains all these nutrients and more within a single cell, some scientists believe that it may have a significant role to play in humanity's future. NASA has conducted studies of chlorella as an ideal food for long-term space travel and colonization. Dr. Dale W. Jenkins of the Office of Space Science and Applications says, "It has been amply demonstrated that chlorella can be used in a closed ecological system to maintain animals such as mice or monkeys. The use of algae for supplying oxygen, food and water and for removing carbon dioxide, water vapor and odors has been considered by many authors for use in spacecraft and space stations, and for establishing bases on the Moon or Mars."

In Third World countries suffering from mass hunger, chlorella may serve as an important food source. It contains four times more protein than eggs and twice as much as chicken, making it a simple, effective way to feed large populations. In underdeveloped countries with poor medical care and sanitary systems, chlorella can help people grow stronger, healthier and less vulnerable to contagion and disease.

Are You Undernourished and Overfed?

In Western countries, the problems are different, but chlorella is equally indispensable. Many people in affluent countries are malnourished from the typical Western diet of highly-processed food grown in depleted soils. Furthermore, our bodies are under constant toxic chemical assault from the environment, including poisons in our food and water. Here chlorella can provide the missing nutrients in our diets, cleanse our systems of toxins and protect us from environmentally-caused cancers.

In recent years, mad cow and hoof-and-mouth disease have contaminated the meat supply that is the staple of the Western diet. These disturbing animal plagues have inspired many people to believe our future diet will be vegetarian. Here, too, chlorella has a major role to play, providing nutrients that are difficult, or even impossible, for vegetarians to obtain.

"No In-Between Meal Cravings..."

One of the most common problems of the typical Western diet is that it leads to obesity. Here is yet another area where chlorella offers health and hope. Many people find that taking chlorella promotes weight loss. The reasons for this are two-fold. First, when you take chlorella, your body is well-nourished, at long last. Hunger pangs and cravings disappear, replaced by a calm satisfaction. Ed Huddle of Aurora, California writes, "I don't seem to have the in-between meal cravings or desire to snack nearly as much as before. And yet, on the other hand, I seem to have more energy than ever!" Without frequent sugar cravings and junk food binges, you may naturally eat fewer calories and, therefore, lose weight.

Another reason you may shed unwanted pounds when you take chlorella is because it fine-tunes your metabolism. With your system cleansed of toxins, your whole body functions more cohesively. Your cells burn more fat and your fluids are released, not retained. An added bonus is that your increased energy can inspire you to exercise, which, of course, is a key to weight control.

And there's no need to worry about the calories in chlorella. At a mere 15 calories per serving (3 grams), chlorella is a guilt-free banquet of pure nutrition!

So Simple, So Miraculous

For all these reasons, chlorella clearly deserves its title of "Superfood for the 21st Century." In one simple package, it delivers the vitamins, minerals and other nutrients that your body urgently needs to stay strong, healthy, clean and youthful. Providing ten times the chlorophyll of spirulina, six times the beta-carotene of spinach, and twice as much protein as steak, chlorella is a food with the power to change our future.

CHAPTER 6
Why Not Stay Young?
How To Keep Strong
and Vital, Year After Year

A wise man once said, "It's not how old you are, but how you are old." We've all marveled at the way some people add on the years, enjoying life, staying physically active and contributing to their communities. For these lucky ones, the later years are truly golden.

But others are not so fortunate. Disease and chronic pain rob them of the chance to participate in their world. Though they struggle valiantly against their increasing limitations, eventually they retreat into a medicated cocoon, frustrated and depressed by all they want to do and can not.

Why do some people age well and others don't? A recent landmark study by the MacArthur Foundation set out to determine the causes. Over a decade, a team of distinguished scientists investigated how we grow old. The resulting book, *Successful Aging*, explains their fascinating conclusions.

Contrary to the popular belief that the secret to aging well is to choose your parents wisely, the MacArthur study emphasizes that what you do has enormous impact on your long-term health. While acknowledging the importance of genetics, the MacArthur study pinpoints three actions you can take to powerfully increase your chances of a vital old age: (1) Exercise regularly. (2) Stay connected to other people. (3) Get the proper nutrition.

Aging And Eating: The Problem Is Real

In the realm of nutrition, chlorella is marvelously equipped to help you meet the challenges of aging. It's an unfortunate fact that as you age, you become more prone to malnutrition. Your metabolism slows down and grows less efficient, thereby rendering your cells less effective at absorbing nutrients. Appetite often decreases, causing you to eat less. And medications can interfere with your food absorption, as well.

The resulting malnutrition can set up a dangerous cycle. Without proper nutritional support, you feel exhausted all the time. This low energy level keeps you from exercising and discourages you from becoming involved in your community: the very things that the MacArthur study says are so important to successful aging. And of course, you grow more vulnerable to disease.

DNA and RNA, The Nucleic Fountain of Youth

If you want to avoid this vicious cycle, chlorella is your ally. According to the late Dr. Benjamin Frank, author of *Dr. Frank's No-Aging Diet*, a diet rich in nucleic acids can powerfully counter the aging process. Chlorella boasts the highest nucleic acid content of any known food. Its dense supply of DNA and RNA allows a single cell of chlorella to regenerate into four new cells every seventeen to twenty hours.

That same regenerative power can go to work on your behalf, revitalizing your energy and putting a long-forgotten spring back in your step. It can ward off painful ailments that sap your joy in living. It can help you sleep at night and keep you mentally alert during the day. And as a wonderful by-product, it can make you look younger too.

Let's take a closer look at chlorella's rejuvenating magic.

"I Have The Energy To Do What I Want To Do"

Increased Vitality: One of the most common experiences that people report when they start taking chlorella is that they feel more energetic. Georgia Alquinta of South Cleelum, Washington writes, "I am 75 years old. Before I started taking chlorella, I had no energy or desire to do anything but sit. Now I walk my dog ten miles every day and have energy to do what I want to do all day. I love this feeling."

Because chlorella nourishes every cell in your body, your whole system starts working more efficiently. Your metabolism gears up to a healthier level; your bowels are cleansed and function better, and your immune system is stimulated. Heavy metals and other toxins are escorted out of your body, lifting a gigantic burden from your system, and promoting delightful new feelings of lightness, well-being and energy.

Freedom From Pain and Illness: Many people who take chlorella discover that chronic conditions from which they suffered for years improve or even disappear. Martha Jones of Santa Maria, California notes that before she took chlorella, "I suffered with chronic bronchitis and digestive problems that kept me worn down. At age 72, I am happy that I now have a healthy digestive system. No more bronchitis or even bursitis."

Other chlorella users have experienced improvements from an astonishing range of ailments. Arthritis sufferer John Garret of Boise, Idaho says that after six months of chlorella, he can walk without a cane.

Virginia Linsteadt of Ukiah, California credits chlorella with curing her sinus headaches, while Carol Cuthill of Fayetteville, North Carolina says it cleared up a persistent skin rash.

How can one health supplement provide relief for so many different ailments? The answer is that chlorella offers a multitude of benefits to the body, working where it is most needed to heal and protect. By rebuilding muscle and tissue, strengthening the immune system and removing damaging toxins, chlorella artfully stimulates the body's own healing powers and puts nature to work on your behalf.

The result is that you may find that chlorella improves your health in many ways, allowing you to enjoy a more active, pain-free life. Tony Hess of Mauston, Wisconsin says, "My blood pressure is normal now, my skin appears healthier, it is easier to breathe now and I rarely feel hungry."

Staying Sharp As A Tack: Brain Food For Brain Power

Heightened Mental Alertness: Chlorella's antioxidants, as well as its revitalizing nucleic acids, are prime factors in the heightened mental powers that many people experience when they take chlorella. Mary Ann Puff of Niagara Falls, New York, age 70, enjoys playing cards with her 73-year-old husband. After six weeks of taking chlorella, she noticed that she now remembers who dealt the last hand and who won the last game. "This seems like a little thing," says Mrs. Puff, "but at my age it is very very important."

A 1989 study of chlorella's effects on patients with Alzheimer's and cerebrovascular dementia showed that it alleviated dementia in 32% and arrested further dementia in 36%! [25] This promising development points the way to chlorella as a powerful brain protector, fighting off the free radical molecules that attack brain cells, causing them to "rust" similar to the same process that rusts metals.

Longer Life: We all want the longest possible life span, but we are not sure how to get it. Taking chlorella can be an important aid in increasing our longevity. Dr. David Steenblock, in his book *Chlorella, Natural Medicinal Algae,* writes that "experiments with laboratory mice have shown that when mice are fed chlorella, their life span can be extended by over 30%."

Chlorella strengthens your immune system, thereby protecting you from lethal diseases that could prematurely end your life. It stimulates your metabolism, so your cells operate with youthful efficiency. And it nourishes your entire body, so you have the zest to engage in life, year after year.

Maybel Jasmund of Edgewater, Florida writes, "My husband had three major surgeries and the doctors have said that his recovery is terrific. People can't believe he is 81; they think he is much younger because he is so full of vitality and strength."

And we can all aspire to the awesome capabilities of devoted chlorella user Frank Ziniker of Saint Petersburg, Florida: "At 97, I do not have aches or pain and work very hard in my small orange grove. I harvest the crop at harvest time on a 16 foot ladder."

A Cycle of Health That Keeps You Young

Nothing we do can stop the calendar, but we can stop helplessly surrendering to the aging process. The MacArthur study urges us to take control of our health in order to enjoy longer, better lives. By taking chlorella, you can start taking control of your nutritional needs and creating a healthy cycle within your body.

When taken on a regular basis, the "green wonder" of chlorella can make you look, feel, and act younger. It can increase your zest for living and your inner peace. And most importantly, it can give you energy that you can share with the world around you.

CHAPTER 7

By Process of Elimination: The Secret of Good Bowel Health

Nobody likes to talk about it, but it's true nonetheless: the key to good health is in your bowels. When your bowels are clean and active, they promptly process digestive waste and eliminate it. But when the bowels are sluggish, they fill with toxins that eventually leak into the bloodstream and spread throughout the body.

A toxic-laden bowel can adversely affect every organ, gland and tissue. Medical researchers at the University of California in San Francisco found that non-nursing women who have less than one bowel movement every three days show significantly more pre-cancerous cells in their breast fluid than women who have one or more bowel movements per day. Dr. Bernard Jensen wrote, "Because the bowel can affect so many other body tissues in this manner without manifesting symptoms itself, we find that heart conditions, liver conditions, lung conditions, kidney conditions and many other conditions are often treated without recognizing and treating the basic source of the problem — a toxic, underactive bowel."

No Warning Signs Till It's Too Late

Sometimes your body sends you signals that your bowels have a problem. You may experience extreme gas, constipation, diarrhea or cramps. But often you receive no warning signs until serious disease, such as cancer, strikes. The reason is simple: the bowel lacks pain-sensitive nerves that could alert you to brewing trouble.

The Western way of life encourages unhealthy bowels. Most of us don't exercise enough, though we should. Exercise improves our digestion and strengthens the functioning of the bowels. An unhealthy diet is the other main culprit. The average American diet consists of 29% wheat and wheat products, 25% milk and milk products and 9% refined sugar, for a total of 63%. Sadly, these items should total 6% of the diet, with the bulk of nutrients coming from fresh fruits, vegetables, proteins and whole grains.

If you are among the millions of people who eat too much of these unhealthy products, you may be interested to know how they affect you. Refined white flour irritates your bowel and coats it with gluten. Excess milk slows down your bowel and causes constipation. And refined sugar contributes to putrefaction in your bowel and overacidity throughout the body.

"After Five Years of Chronic and Serious Constipation..."

What should you eat to promote good bowel health? One of the best bowel stimulants is fiber, an indigestible vegetable cellulose. In the words of Dr. Jensen, fiber "tones and exercises the bowel wall, absorbs moisture and decreases bowel transit time."

You can add fiber to your diet by eating lots of fresh fruit, vegetables and whole grains. You can also enrich your fiber intake with chlorella. Chlorella's dietary fibers work in tandem with its other nutrients to strengthen and cleanse the bowel, often with remarkable results.

"Chlorella has done wonders for me in only a couple of months," writes Dorothy Scott of San Angelo, Texas. "I always had to take a laxative before and now I don't have this problem." Susan Stephan of Saint Petersburg, Florida comments, "After five years of chronic and serious constipation, after years of laxatives and herbs and chemicals, and finally after a colonoscopy to look for possible cancer, I found a complete and unexpected healing from chlorella tablets! It is still a bit of a thrill, after nearly a year, to have a daily bowel movement and still a bit of a surprise. It has, no doubt, helped me to save my life — and I am only 38!"

Four Ingredients Working In Harmony

The fiber in chlorella is one of four components that join together to detoxify your bowel. Chlorophyll, the most powerful cleansing agent in nature, swiftly goes to work, eliminating trapped toxins. "As it begins to detoxify the bowel, it also detoxifies the liver and bloodstream, feeds the friendly bowel flora and soothes irritated tissue along the bowel wall," wrote Dr. Jensen. Chlorella Growth Factor (CGF) provides ample healing nutrients for the bowel wall, while chlorella's high protein content assists in repairing and rebuilding damaged tissue.

An important aspect of chlorella's success in the bowel is that it promotes "friendly" flora and eliminates damaging ones. The average colon contains 400 to 500 species of bacteria, fungi, yeast and viruses. Some of them, like lactobacillus acidophilus, are marvelous aids in the digestive process, helping to form the B-vitamins. Chlorella encourages these beneficial flora to flourish. But other species, such as E. Coli, are dangerous disease-mongers that multiply with frightening rapidity. Here's where chlorella's powers come to the rescue, battling these nasty flora and removing their poisonous wastes from your system.

Chlorella for Sweeter Smells

Over the years, clinical studies have documented chlorella's beneficial effect on the bowel. A 1980 experiment by Drs. Young and Beregi found that chlorophyll relieved chronic constipation problems in nursing home patients. Additionally, in 85% of the cases, a noticeable relief of intestinal gas in terms of amount and odor was observed.

Chlorophyll is legendary for its deodorizing abilities, and has long been used as an underarm deodorant and to control bad breath. These beneficial effects on smell also apply to the bowel area. Drs. Young and Beregi state, "It is common knowledge among workers in nursing homes, geriatric hospitals and mental institutions that chlorophyllin is an important aid in the control of odors from incontinent patients." And in 1951, Drs. Weingarten and Payson found a significant reduction of odor in patients with colostomies when they were administered a daily dose of chlorophyllin. [26]

What's Good For Your Bowel Is Good For Your Body

To protect your health, you need a clean, active bowel. You need to insure that waste products are promptly eliminated, instead of lingering, putrefying and spreading into your blood stream. That's why chlorella is a blessing to your elimination process. In the words of the late Dr. Bernard Jensen, "Chlorella raises tissue to its optimal level of integrity when taken consistently over a long period of time, helping correct mineral deficiencies, remove toxic accumulations and repair damaged tissue…We can't rebuild a toxic bowel overnight, but we can make a healthy start."

CHAPTER 8

Good as New: Repairing Tissue and Healing Wounds

The patient was in despair. Her legs were covered with 13 open ulcers, some the size of silver dollars. For three years, she had sought help, but even the leading medical clinics had been unable to cure her. In her misery, she turned to a young doctor who was beginning to study the connection between nutrition and health. He decided to try the healing power of chlorophyll, the green "lifeblood" of plants.

The young doctor chopped up the green tops of nine different vegetables. He soaked them in water, strained them and gave three to four quarts of this "concentrated sunshine" to his patient to drink, every day for three weeks. The results shocked both patient and doctor: all 13 leg ulcers vanished.

From that moment on, the doctor, Bernard Jensen, devoted himself to finding more effective ways to deliver chlorophyll. He investigated many different kinds of algae before finding the species that he wanted. "There are 25,000 forms of algae," wrote Dr. Jensen. "Chlorella is the best of them all."

Before Antibiotics, The Miracle of Chlorophyll

Chlorella contains more chlorophyll than any known plant. This important fact helps explain why chlorella has proved so successful at healing ulcers and wounds. Before our modern era of "wonder drugs" and antibiotics, chlorophyll was touted by scientists as a miraculously effective repair agent of tissue. In their excitement about chlorophyll's powers, scientists conducted a multitude of studies:

In 1930, the *American Journal of Surgery* published an article which made headlines around the world. Doctors at Temple University had treated over 1,200 patients, suffering from a wide variety of ailments, with chlorophyll. According to Dr. Jensen, "Chlorophyll diluted with sterile water was used to clean out deep surgical wounds, some of them badly infected. Ulcerated varicose veins, osteomyelitis, brain ulcers and shallow, open wounds were cleansed with chlorophyll solution or covered with a chlorophyll salve. Diseases of the mouth, such as trench-mouth and advanced pyorhhea, were treated. The results were spectacular. The doctors who tested the chlorophyll hailed it as an important and effective therapy." [27]

In 1944, five hundred tissue cultures were grown. When chlorophyll was added to the cultures, they showed well-defined growth within six to eight hours, unlike the control group. Initial signs of tissue growth were apparent within two hours. [28]

Ulcer and Wounds Cured By Chlorella

After World War II, antibiotics became the focus of mainstream medicine for healing wounds and ulcers. Yet the following study shows how antibiotics can benefit when coupled with the healing power of chlorophyll. In a 1945 experiment, chlorophyll was given for infected ulcers. When chlorophyll was used in combination with penicillin, the healing rate of wounds increased by 35% over the use of either penicillin or chlorophyll by itself. [29]

And despite the magnificent record of antibiotics and other modern drugs, they don't always provide healing. Some patients suffer from wounds and ulcers that refuse to respond to them. That's why the following experiments are of immense importance to people in need of tissue rejuvenation:

At Saito Hospital in Japan, doctors gave chlorella to patients with stomach and duodenal ulcers who were not responding to the usual medications. In most of the patients, the pain vanished within ten days of taking three grams daily of chlorella. Within 21 to 40 days, most other symptoms disappeared. X-rays showed the ulcers had completely healed in most cases, and a miniature medical camera proved that new tissue had closed up the ulcers. [30]

Chlorella tablets and a chlorella extract in tablet form were given to patients with chronic wounds that failed to respond satisfactorily to standard medications. All the patients soon achieved improvements and new skin formation. [31]

"Chlorella Often Offers Immediate Results..."

Dr. David Steenblock often gives chlorella to patients who suffer from ulcers. In addition to chlorella's high chloropyll content, he credits its nucleic acids with the ability to promote tissue repair. Dr. Steenblock uses the liquid extract of Chlorella Growth Factor (CGF), which contains a high concentration of the nucleic acids RNA and DNA, for healing both internal and external ulcers.

"The CGF liquid can be very beneficial to conditions of the upper intestinal tract such as an irritated esophagus or stomach ulcers," according to Dr. Steenblock. "This is because of the direct soothing and healing effects upon the tissues from the concentrations of CGF. The chlorella liquid extract often offers immediate results in such upper intestinal tract problems. The liquid CGF also has topical applications for skin conditions such as diabetic ulcers."

Dr. Steenblock notes that the healing of skin ulcers depends on a certain kind of cell called a fibroblast. Chlorella aids the production and growth of fibroblasts. "This may be one of the reasons that chlorella promotes the healing of skin ulcers so rapidly," said Dr. Steenblock.

A Natural Path to Healing

In the modern world of "wonder drugs" and antibiotics, chlorella offers an additional, natural path to healing. Its high chlorophyll content gives you the restorative power of "concentrated sunshine," while its nucleic acids swiftly stimulate your body's own healing powers. If you suffer from chronic ulcers or wounds, chlorella's nutrients can bring your damaged tissues a whole new lease on life.

CHAPTER 9

Good Heart Health: Controlling High Blood Pressure and Cholesterol

Every 33 seconds, an American dies of cardiovascular disease. Heart disease is the leading killer in the United States, claiming more lives each year than the next six leading causes of death combined. Many women fear cancer as their most likely killer, yet 53% of women die of heart disease. In fact, heart disease annually claims the lives of 504,000 women; in comparison, breast cancer claims the lives of 42,000.

In a culture in which heart disease has reached such staggering proportions, what can you do to protect your health? For guidance, it's instructive to turn to the American Heart Association, which advises that the best way to avoid heart disease is to eat a healthy diet. Recently, the Association published a new set of dietary guidelines, designed to be easier to use and which stresses overall eating patterns, instead of avoidance of fats.

"We are emphasizing the positive message of what people should eat - for example, more plant-based foods," says Robert M. Krauss, M.D., principal author of the dietary guidelines. "In the past, we have focused rather heavily on the percentage of calories as fat and amounts of cholesterol. These are still important considerations, but the emphasis has shifted to allow consumers to understand the importance of an overall eating plan."

How To Eat A Heart-Healthy Diet

If you are interested in following the American Heart Association dietary guidelines, chlorella can help you do just that. The Association advocates eating a balanced diet rich in plant-based foods. Chlorella provides you with a wide range of plant-based vitamins, minerals, amino acids, and omega fatty acids that strongly support and supplement your nutritional choices.

Furthermore, a wealth of clinical data proves that chlorella, when taken on a regular basis, can dramatically improve your heart health. Dr. Bernard Jensen noted, "There is persuasive evidence that high blood pressure, high triglycerides and high cholesterol are lowered by regular use of chlorella." From preventing plaque build-up to increasing the elasticity of arteries, chlorella gets to the heart of the matter, improving your cardio-vascular functioning and protecting you from dangerous heart diseases.

Reducing Cholesterol Levels With Chlorella

For example, let's take a look at chlorella and its effect on high cho-lesterol. When present in excess, cholesterol tends to stick to artery walls, creating a dangerous buildup of fat. As the artery walls thicken and hard-en, they drive up blood pressure and cause serious stresses on the heart.

Chlorella can effectively go to work reducing high cholesterol levels. In a pilot study in Japan, patients took 9 grams of chlorella every day for a year, making no other changes in their diet. The researchers found that cholesterol levels were "significantly" lowered in these chlorella users. [32] A recent study in the United States documented similar results. [33]

Another experiment involved rabbits that were fed a high-cholesterol diet. When a 1% chlorella powder was added to their menu, the rabbits' cholesterol level improved, and the lesions on their aorta were reduced by two-thirds. Chlorella's effect surpassed the cholesterol-lowering drug Clofibrate, which was used as a control. [34] (figure 4)

One problem with high cholesterol levels is that they harden the artery walls, making them less flexible. This, in turn, forces the heart to pump harder. In his book, *Chlorella: Natural Medicinal Algae*, Dr. David Steenblock describes an experiment in which patients were given a very small dose of chlorella for two months. Half of the participants showed improved blood vessel elasticity. Dr. Steenblock notes that future studies of longer duration and higher doses of chlorella may well deliver even more dramatic results. [35]

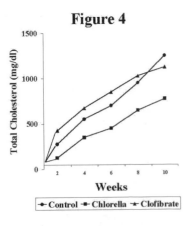

Figure 4

Effect of powdered chlorella or Clofibrate on the level of total choles-terol in serum in cholesterol-fed rabbits.

High Blood Pressure: Danger Ahead!

The American way of life — a high-fat diet and a sedentary lifestyle — creates the perfect conditions for high blood pressure. In fact, 50 mil-lion Americans have hypertension (high blood pressure), putting them at risk for kidney disease, stroke, heart attack and heart failure. Unfortunately, many people with high blood pressure do not realize they have it, because doctors often do not warn patients until their levels climb to dangerous extremes. A 1999 study indicated that 39% of people with high blood pressure did not realize that they had it; 16% were not being treated adequately and 28% were unable to control their problem. [36]

If you have high blood pressure, or are at risk for developing high blood pressure, you should know that chlorella can help you gain control of this serious condition. A joint study by American and Japanese scientists evaluated the effects of chlorella extract on rats with extremely high blood pressure. On average, the rats' blood pressure dropped 20 mm Hg after three hours. [37]

Another intriguing study indicated that people with mild to moderate hypertension may be able to control their levels with chlorella alone. Patients took ten grams of chlorella and three ounces of liquid extract and stopped using their blood pressure medications. Thirty-eight percent of the patients showed some improvement in hypertension with chlorella supplementation. When analyzed using a smaller scale of change, almost half of the patients showed as good or better results than they did with medications. [33]

Smoking Is Hazardous To Your Heart

Smoking devastates your cardiovascular system. If you are a smoker, the single best move you can make for your health and your loved ones' health, is to stop smoking. That's because when you smoke, you not only inflict terrible damage on your own heart, you also assault the hearts of the people around you. Non-smokers who live with heavy smokers have four times the risk of heart attack as people living in a smoke-free home.

Cigarette smoke causes hardening of the arteries and encourages the formation of dangerous blood clots. It compromises delivery of oxygen to the heart and reduces the heart's functioning. Its cumulative effect on every system of the body is overwhelmingly toxic.

If you can't stop smoking, or if you live in a home where someone else smokes, chlorella can offer you at least some measure of protection. Cigarette smoke contains cadmium, a heavy metal associated with high blood pressure, blood clotting and hardening of the arteries. Chlorella is a remarkably effective natural cleanser of cadmium, removing it from the body safely and swiftly. Japanese patients who were suffering from cadmium poisoning were given chlorella daily for 24 days. After 12 days, their rate of cadmium excretion had tripled. After 24 days, their excretion rate had increased seven times. [38] This encouraging evidence shows that chlorella can help you remove the toxic residue of smoking from your body, instead of letting it linger and create heart-rending damage.

Getting To The Heart of the Matter

Sixty million Americans suffer from one or more forms of cardiovascular disease. With heart disease as the nation's leading killer, we should all take special care of our hearts. That means adding moderate exercise to our daily routine, not smoking, and following the American Heart Association's recommendations to eat a balanced diet rich in plant-based foods.

Chlorella can be an important part of that diet. It nourishes you with plant-based nutrients that are clinically proven to lower high blood pressure, prevent hardening of the arteries and reduce cholesterol. One of the most powerful steps you can take for your health is to protect your heart with chlorella.

CHAPTER 10
Alzheimer's Disease: A Nutritional Approach

The facts are heart-breaking: over 4 million Americans suffer from Alzheimer's disease, a slow death of the brain. Among people who live to 85, fully half will suffer from this devastating illness, which kills off neurons deep within the brain that regulate memory and cognition.

As Alzheimer's sufferers descend into a morass of confusion, depression and psychosis, the burden of caring for them falls on their loved ones. Seventy percent of Alzheimer's patients live with their families, placing a gigantic strain upon these caregivers who must cope with the gradual destruction of someone they love.

What can you do to protect yourself from this increasingly-common disease? How can you help someone who is already suffering from Alzheimer's to reverse their helpless downward slide?

The Nutrients You Need For Brain Health

As scientists investigate a variety of promising approaches, a new emphasis on brain health through nutrition has emerged. In *The Brain Wellness Plan*, Drs. Jay Lombard and Carl Germano suggest that you can begin now, "no matter what your age - to add the nutrients so essential to supporting brain health and a vital brain-immune connection."

In this new nutritional approach to brain health, chlorella may be destined to play a vital role. A Japanese study shows that chlorella can significantly improve symptoms of dementia. A group of patients suffering from cerebrovascular dementia or Alzheimer's was given chlorella extract and tablets. Thirty-two percent showed signs of alleviated dementia and 36% stopped developing further dementia. [25]

Alzheimer's and Heavy Metals: What's The Real Story?

Although we have much to learn about Alzheimer's, we can make some general observations about why chlorella can be effective in both its prevention and treatment.

One school of thought holds that Alzheimer's is related to heavy metal exposure. Higher levels of various heavy metals have been found in the brains and blood of patients with Alzheimer's, but the link with

Alzheimer's remains controversial.

Whatever its ultimate role in causing Alzheimer's, heavy metals such as aluminum and mercury are well-known neurotoxins, which disrupt more than 50 chemical reactions in your body. Limiting your exposure to heavy metals is a wise choice. So is removing them from your system with chlorella. Chlorella contains chlorophyll, which is well-documented as a supremely effective remover of heavy metal toxins from the body. As scientists debate the exact linkage of these toxins and Alzheimer's, you can help protect your brain by safely escorting them out of your system with chlorella.

B Well, B Brain Healthy

The B vitamins are key players in brain wellness, and an increasing number of studies have connected Alzheimer's to vitamin B deficiencies. Alzheimer's patients have shown seriously low levels of vitamin B-12 in their cerebrospinal fluid. Other tests have exposed the link between Alzheimer's and low levels of thiamine (vitamin B-1), including a study reported in *Annals of Neurology* in which Alzheimer's patients treated with B-1 showed marked improvement. [39]

This correlation between the B vitamins and Alzheimer's is another important clue in understanding chlorella's beneficial impact on brain health. Chlorella contains an abundance of B vitamins, including thiamine (B-1), riboflavin (B-2), pyridoxine (B-6) and more vitamin B-12 than beef liver.

Fighting Free Radicals That Attack Your Brain

A recent Canadian study provided fascinating insight into the workings of Alzheimer's: samples of Alzheimer's brain tissue showed nearly 50 percent more free radicals than the control samples. [40] Free radicals are short-lived molecules which rampage through your body, attacking cell membranes and genetic codes, and unleashing the forces of aging.

The best way to fight free radicals is with antioxidants. These nutrients disarm the arsenal of free radicals, and prevent them from spreading cell damage in your brain. Chlorella contains potent antioxidants, such as carotenoids, that protect your brain from vicious attacks by free radical "terrorists."

One unfortunate effect of free radicals is that they inflame the brain, a condition associated with Alzheimer's. Essential fatty acids are excellent anti-inflammatory agents, reducing inflammation and preventing its recurrence. Chlorella offers the complete spectrum of essential fatty acids, promoting good brain health by fighting swelling of the brain and supporting optimum communication between nerve cells.

Here's Some Food for Thought

Along with all the nutrients already mentioned, chlorella contains a host of other ingredients recommended in *The Brain Wellness Plan*. It's a rich supplier of zinc, which is an essential element for brain functions. In fact, some scientists believe a deficiency of zinc causes Alzheimer's. And it teems with nucleic acids, which stimulate the immune system to protect you from free radicals.

The good news is that progress is being made in the war against Alzheimer's disease, as scientists explore vaccines and probe its genetic basis. In the meantime, until a cure-all is here, you can supply your brain with the nutrients it needs to stay alert and active. Taking chlorella is smart thinking for a healthy brain.

CHAPTER 11
Cold, Flu and Viral Infections

One of the most common changes that people report once they start taking chlorella is that they no longer "catch every bug." Even during the height of cold and flu season, they seem to remain invulnerable, happily going about their business while other people take to their beds, coughing and sneezing. And, if they do catch a cold, its symptoms are milder and they can shake it off sooner than they did before taking chlorella.

"Every year everyone in my office gets some major flu or infection and I still have to work closely with them, but I have never caught their illnesses," says William Porter of Los Angeles, California. "I believe it's the chlorella that has strengthened my immune system. If I have felt a cold coming on, I increase my use of chlorella and it has always worked to prevent a cold."

Mary Schindler of Beloit, Wisconsin notes, "My husband and I began taking chlorella about four years ago when he retired. I have many allergies and in the past, a cold would hang on for a month or more, even though I took vitamins for years previously. I have not had a cold in four years. For me this is a miracle! He would not want to be without chlorella! Neither of us has been sick."

200 Viruses Can Cause A Cold

Chlorella's ability to protect you from colds and other viral infections is good news indeed, because exposure to these germs is everywhere. Over 200 different viruses can cause a cold, and their collective impact creates one billion colds a year in the United States alone. Children are most prone to colds: school-age children contract up to twelve colds a year. Adults average two to four colds a year, with women more prone to them than men.

Flu, which is caused by the influenza virus, causes symptoms similar to colds, although it tends to come on suddenly. The flu can be fatal to older people, young children and people with chronic illnesses. In fact, 20,000 people die every year from influenza.

Impossible Advice: Don't Breathe!

Fortunately, a flu vaccine does exist, and people who are in a high-risk category should be vaccinated every year. But despite the massive research into creating a cold vaccine, no prospect is in sight. Developing a vaccine that can fight off 200 different viruses is still too complex for modern science.

Therefore, prevention is your best bet for avoiding viral infections. Doctors advise washing your hands frequently, using disinfectants on household surfaces and avoiding exposure to people with colds. Viruses can hang in the air, waiting to be inhaled by new victims, so not breathing the air around contaminated people is wise — and just about impossible. Infected people are everywhere, and the best you can hope for is to limit exposure, not prevent it altogether.

The Good News From Japanese Sailors

That's why chlorella is such good news for people who are prone to catching seasonal illnesses and viral infections. Its nutrients offer you much-needed protection, stimulating your immune system and powerfully strengthening your ability to fight off troublesome viral invaders.

Interesting evidence of chlorella's cold-fighting powers comes from a clinical trial of 971 Japanese sailors. During a long, grueling assignment at sea, 458 sailors took chlorella. These sailors had 26% fewer colds than sailors in the control group. [1] And, in a 1990 study at the Medical College of Virginia, chlorella was given to patients with suppressed immune systems as a result of having tumors. These patients showed near-normal levels of immune system function and experienced fewer respiratory infections and flu-like illnesses than patients in the control group. [5]

"Not A Single Case in Which Improvement or Cure Has Not Taken Place"

If you do have the misfortune to contract a cold or viral illness, chlorella can help you bounce back quicker. Tami Polinar of Gardena, California says that now when she gets sick, "my colds, for example, last about two days. Usually they last a week and a half. Doctors can't do anything for your cold, but chlorella honestly gets rid of it."

This phenomenon was noted on a massive scale by Drs. Ridpath and Davis, who administered chlorophyll packs to over 1,000 cases of respiratory infections, sinusitis and head colds. The doctors reported, "There is not a single case in which improvement or cure has not taken place." Chlorophyll packs placed on sinuses vastly improved symptoms, and head colds tended to disappear within 24 hours.

Recipe for Relief: Clear up Congestion with Chlorella

In his book, *Chlorella, Natural Medicinal Algae*, Dr. David Steenblock offers a chlorophyll-rich remedy for congested sinuses and nostrils:

Salt Water Nasal Wash for Sinusitis and Nasal Congestion

✔ Add ½ teaspoon table salt to 1 pint lukewarm water

✔ Place solution in soup bowl.

✔ Over sink, block one nostril from side with index finger.

✔ Dip nose into solution and inhale through nose to bring liquid into mouth.

✔ Remove bowl from under nose and allow solution to drain from nose and mouth.

✔ Repeat until ½ solution is used per nostril.

Dr. Steenblock writes, "This standard remedy for congested sinuses and nostrils may be modified by boiling 3 grams of chlorella (1 packet granules or 1 teaspoon powder per pint water), strain through cheese cloth while hot and then use as described above (i.e., add the salt to this pint of water + chlorella).

Stay Healthy and Happy During Cold and Flu Season

If you want to remain healthy and active, even during the fall and winter months when colds and flu abound, chlorella is your little green ally. It can strengthen your immune system so you fight off the viral invaders that lurk in the air, on doorknobs, towels, phones, handrails, desks and just about anyplace else.

If you have children in the family, you can help them avoid the frequent illnesses passed around their classroom by fortifying them with chlorella. And you can protect the rest of the family from the illnesses that the children bring home by giving them chlorella too.

Then perhaps everyone in the family can be as blessed as Harry Dunham of Mooresville, Indiana: "I have faithfully taken chlorella for approximately three years. I have not encountered any illness, not even a minor cold during this time. I am 75 years of age, employed part time by a major firm and have no lost time due to illness."

CHAPTER 12
New Approaches To Fibromyalgia

If you suffer from fibromyalgia, you know what a nightmare this illness can be. You wake up stiff, tired and throbbing with pain. Your muscles and joints ache all day, exhausting you, and turning the simplest task into a gigantic undertaking. Even a visit to the bathroom can be a painful trial. At the end of a long torturous day, you climb stiffly into bed, hoping for sleep. Instead, you find yourself tossing and turning for hours, aching and anxious.

Fibromyalgia, formerly known as fibrositis, is a syndrome that causes chronic pain in muscles, joints, ligaments and the tissue that surrounds them, as well as extreme fatigue, sleep problems, depression, bowel problems and other symptoms. Seven times more common in women than men, fibromyalgia can be found in 3 to 6% of the United States population. Although you can get fibromyalgia at any age, it strikes most often between the ages of 20 and 40.

For many years, the medical establishment did not officially recognize fibromyalgia. However, in 1991, The American College of Rheumatology finally defined this incapacitating syndrome. There are eighteen "tender points" on the body, and if a patient has pain when touched at eleven or more, a diagnosis of fibromyalgia can be made.

What Causes Fibromyalgia?

Although fibromyalgia has been the subject of much recent research, its cause remains elusive. Some scientists believe an infectious virus is to blame; so far, this theory has no proof. Other researchers contend that injury or trauma to the central nervous system sets off the disease, while still others believe it is caused by problems with muscle metabolism.

For now, standard treatment consists of a combination of exercise, medication (including anti-depressants), physical therapy and relaxation. Many patients find some relief from these approaches, but often the relief is limited and temporary. The disease remains extraordinarily frustrating for those who suffer from it, massively disrupting their ability to concentrate, work and enjoy life.

Recent Studies Show Chlorella
Eases Fibromyalgia Symptoms

If you suffer from fibromyalgia, you may frequently feel hopeless. That's why it's important you know that two recent studies suggest chlorella can significantly ease fibromyalgia symptoms. In an initial study, 18 patients took 50 tablets (10g) of chlorella and 100 ml. of chlorella liquid extract daily for two months. Nearly all the patients in this initial study reported that taking chlorella relieved some of their pain, stabilized their body functions and generally improved the quality of their daily life.

Based on these encouraging results, a team of physicians led by Dr. Randall Merchant of the Medical College of Virginia, designed a second, more extensive study of the effect of chlorella on fibromyalgia. In this study of 34 patients, half were put on a regimen of 50 tablets of chlorella and 100 ml. of chlorella liquid daily for three months. The other half of the group was given placebo tablets and liquid. After the initial three-month period, and a "washout" period of one month, the two groups were switched.

Remarkably, 62 % of the patients taking chlorella reported an average drop of 31% in their pain. The placebo group reported an 8% drop. The patients taking chlorella also slept better, experienced more energy and felt less anxiety. [33]

"I'm Able To Take Really Goods Walks Now"

Let's meet two of the participants in this landmark study. Ena Van Rooyen had been suffering from aching joints, sleeplessness and tension headaches for more than 20 years. She was a member of the group that received chlorella first. Six weeks into the study, Ena realized her fatigue and pain had gone away. But, as soon as she switched and started taking the placebo, her symptoms returned. On the basis of these heartening results, Ena began taking chlorella on her own.

"I'm able to take really good walks now," says Ena, "and I'm traveling better. I'm also not nearly as forgetful as I used to be. I'm sleeping somewhat better, and I'm hopeful that I'll continue to improve daily."

"Always Felt Like I Was Moving Through Mud"

Stressful situations or trauma to the body may trigger fibromyalgia. In Deborah Donati's case, her symptoms became truly unbearable after a Caesarean section. She experienced constant pain, muscle weakness, numbness in her arms and legs, exhaustion and badly disturbed sleep.

"I always felt like I was moving through mud," Deborah reported. "It was so frustrating. I could never get accomplished what I wanted to get accomplished in a day."

While Deborah took chlorella, she felt more energy, less pain and a heightened sense of well-being. She even began to sleep well for the first time in years. When she went on the placebo, however, her symptoms quickly returned, worse than ever.

Deborah now takes chlorella on her own and reports that she has less pain, renewed energy and more restful sleep.

New Hope, New Approaches For Fibromyalgia Sufferers

As researchers delve into new ways to relieve this debilitating disease, fibromyalgia patients can add chlorella to their repertoire of remedies. Used in tandem with medication, exercise and physical therapy, chlorella can powerfully ease symptoms and help fibromyalgia sufferers rediscover the joy in life.

CHAPTER 13
Keeping Your Liver Healthy

Consider the liver. Weighing in at 2½ to 3½ pounds, the liver is the largest organ in the body and also one of the busiest. It constantly performs thousands of functions, including the removal of toxins from the body and bacteria from the blood, the storage of vitamins, minerals, iron and sugars, the control of production of cholesterol, and the preparation of nutrients in the blood for assimilation by the cells.

According to the late Dr. Bernard Jensen, "The liver is a kind of one-man band in the body…In fact, the liver does so many things, it is subject to breakdown in more ways than most organs, and liver breakdown or underactivity affects every single organ and every single tissue in the body."

A Dangerous Job…But Some Organ Has Got To Do It!

As the detoxifying center of the body, the liver performs a highly dangerous job. A never-ending barrage of poisons arrives for filtering: chemical food additives, bacterial wastes, incompletely digested proteins, pesticides, heavy metals, toxins formed in the bowel, and in some people, alcohol and drugs.

A healthy liver can keep up the pace. But a liver that is sluggish and overwhelmed will eventually allow poisons to infiltrate the bloodstream. From there, the toxins will be carried to every organ, gland and tissue in the body, sowing the seeds of serious disease.

How Can You Treat Your Liver Right?

You need to be good to your liver, so your liver will be good to you. Of course, one of the most important actions you can take for good liver health is to limit your consumption of alcohol. Excess alcohol leads to cirrhosis, a potentially fatal disease in which scar tissue in the liver blocks veins and causes organ failure.

In addition to moderating your alcohol intake, you should eat a healthy diet. "The health of the liver depends on what is going on behind the scenes in the lungs, stomach, pancreas and bowel, day by day, year by year. A continuing poor diet and a chronically underactive bowel wear down the liver as the constant dripping of water wears away rock," wrote Dr. Jensen. "What good would it do to treat the liver if the diet remained unchanged?"

Chlorella, Your Liver's Green Friend

One of the most effective ways to be good to your liver is to supplement your diet with chlorella. A number of important studies document chlorella's beneficial effects on liver health.

In Germany, Dr. Hermann Fink compared the effects of algae on the liver with that of other foods. Rats fed an all-skim milk diet died of liver disease. Almost all the rats fed only egg whites also died of liver disease. But all the rats who were fed only algae remained healthy. [41]

A more recent experiment examined the impact of chlorella in protecting the liver from ethionine, a toxic chemical. Rats who were given a 5% chlorella supplementation in their diets showed less liver damage than the control group and recovered faster. The researchers concluded that even low levels of chlorella supplementation protects the liver from damage due to malnutrition or toxins. [42]

Dr. Jensen explained how chlorella builds and restores liver health: "Chlorella rescues a toxin-laden, fatty, mineral-deficient liver by a combination of methods. First, its chlorophyll cleanses and soothes the irritated tissue in the bowel and builds up the hemoglobin content of the blood. Secondly, chlorella stimulates better bowel function and increased bowel elimination, as noted in Japanese and U.S. medical studies. Better bowel function carries off more cholesterol and fats in the waste, instead of becoming more of a problem. Further, the high DNA/RNA content of chlorella directly stimulates liver tissue repair at the cellular level."

Cirrhosis and Chlorella:
"My Liver Function Tests Stabilized"

Chlorella's health-building powers can even help improve symptoms of cirrhosis, a notoriously difficult-to-treat disease. In *Chlorella: Jewel of the Far East*, Dr. Jensen quoted a 49-year-old man who was hospitalized for alcoholic cirrhosis: "I began taking 30 chlorella tablets (6 grams) a day along with CGF (chlorella growth factor) liquid. For three or four months, there was little effect, and then my liver function tests stabilized at low-normal levels."

Dr. Jensen also quoted a 76-year-old man: "In 1979, I was hospitalized on account of cirrhosis of the liver and diabetes (for nine months). After being discharged, I continued to receive treatment. In 1981, I began to take 40 chlorella tablets daily, together with CGF. My physical condition improved day by day. Now I do not tire no matter what work I do."

Hepatitis C, The Viral Contagion

In recent years, the plague of hepatitis C has increasingly come to the public's attention. Four million Americans suffer from this liver disease, which is caused by a contagious virus in the blood. Hepatitis C is spread by contact with the blood of an infected person, either through a blood transfusion, or from such activities as tattooing, body piercing or sharing needles for drugs.

Hepatitis C causes serious liver damage, including swelling and scarring that can eventually lead to liver failure. Treatment for hepatitis C includes the administration of interferon, a protein naturally produced by the body to protect itself from viral infections. It is interesting to note that chlorella boosts interferon production in the body, as proven in a number of clinical experiments.

A Healthy Liver Makes For A Healthy Body

An active, high-functioning liver helps every organ of your body maintain its peak health. By taking chlorella on a regular basis, you can support the myriad functions your liver must perform to keep you healthy and happy, year in and year out.

CHAPTER 14
Easing The Misery of Allergies and Chemical Sensitivities

W hat causes allergies? Why do some people break out in hives when they eat berries, get sneezing fits when they're near a cat, or become red-eyed and congested during pollen season?

The answer lies in the confusion of the immune system. Primed to combat dangerous invaders, the immune system mistakes a harmless substance such as cat hairs for a serious threat and goes on the attack. First, it releases an allergy-fighting antibody called immunoglobulin E, or IgE. Then, IgE persuades other cells to barrage the allergen with powerful chemicals called histamines. Unfortunately, histamines can set off serious allergic reactions, including rashes, wheezing, hay fever, bronchitis, vomiting, eczema, asthma, swelling and migraine headaches.

Different Allergies, Different Reactions

There are several different types of allergies, and some people suffer from more than one kind. Respiratory allergies can be set off by inhaled substances such as pollen, dust, mold and animal dander. Typically, these allergies result in inflammation and swelling of the delicate lining of the nose, sinuses and eyelids, violent sneezing, nasal congestion, itchy throat and runny eyes. Asthma is a severe reaction to inhaled allergens, in which the air passages narrow, breathing becomes difficult and an attack of wheezing occurs.

Food allergies can be difficult to diagnose, because their symptoms can mimic other problems, such as irritable bowel syndrome or food intolerance. These symptoms can range from diarrhea to abdominal pain, cramps, facial swelling, vomiting, eczema and hives. Some common food culprits are milk, eggs, nuts, fish, chocolate, wheat and corn. Fortunately, if you are allergic to a food, there's an excellent chance you'll outgrow it.

The Secret Allergy You May Be Suffering From

Many people are allergic to every-day materials and don't realize it. They suffer from sensitivities to chemicals such as formaldehyde, chlorine and carbolic acid or metals like nickel, mercury and beryllium. People who work with these substances on their job are more prone to developing allergies to them, but you can develop an allergy from exposure at home, too. Diagnosing exactly which chemical or metal you are allergic to is a tricky proposition. Avoiding contact with the offending substance can be even trickier, if not downright impossible, because some of these chemicals are in hundreds of household items from furniture to carpeting to permanent-press clothing.

"Chlorella May Be Useful For Prevention of Allergic Diseases"

If you suffer from allergies or suspect that you may be susceptible, you will be interested to know that many chlorella users report that they find a significant easing of symptoms.

Rita Free of Tampa Bay, Florida has a young daughter with severe allergies. Since taking chlorella, she writes, "The difference in Angela is tremendous...After taking chlorella 10 months, she is more alert, active and growing by leaps and bounds...In the last two months, Angela has started taking dancing lessons, joined Girl Scouts and started roller skating. She had no interest in these before."

Chlorella contains chlorophyll, the most powerful detoxifying agent in nature. This fact helps explain why chlorella can ease allergic reactions, including those of chemical sensitivities. Chlorella binds to heavy metals and other toxins and safely removes these allergic irritants from your system.

Figure 5

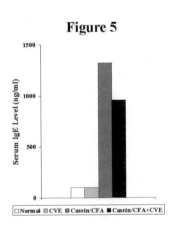

Casein-specific IgE levels in serum from mice which were immunized with casein in CFA. Chow containing 2% chlorella extract (CVE) was given to mice for 2 weeks before casein injection and was also given after injection throughout the experiments. Blood samples were obtained from mice 3 weeks after casein/CFA injection.

In addition, a fascinating study shows that chlorella may limit the production of immunoglobulin E (IgE), the antibody to blame for setting off the allergic chain reaction in your body. In this study, mice who received chlorella extract showed suppressed production of IgE against milk. The researchers concluded that chlorella could be useful in the prevention of certain allergic diseases. [43] (figure 5)

A recent study in Japan explored

chlorella's impact on children with bronchial asthma and a related skin rash. Over 60% of children given three to five grams daily for six months showed improvement. The children's response to food allergens was also notably improved. [44]

An Allergy Strategy Should Include Chlorella

Life with allergies can be challenging. Whether you suffer from respiratory allergies, chemical sensitivities or food allergies, you are forced to deal with a host of unpleasant, exhausting symptoms.

Your doctor can help you develop a health regimen to cope with your allergies that may include medications and immunization. You can also add chlorella to your strategy, so you can reap the rewards of its allergy-fighting nutrients. Even during the height of allergy season, you can feel healthier, stronger and breathe easier with chlorella.

CHAPTER 15
Cancer Prevention and Treatment

Cancer. The very word sends a chill down the spine. Probably the disease that people fear most, cancer can only be treated with severely debilitating procedures that pose serious risks of their own.

If you or a loved one is facing the challenge of surgery, chemotherapy and radiation, there is urgent information you must know: chlorella may offer you invaluable assistance every step of the way.

Let's look at some of the compelling scientific evidence on chlorella's ability to support and stimulate the immune system as it fights cancer.

Easing The Trauma of Chemotherapy

Chemotherapy is built on a contradiction: it destroys cancer cells, but it also destroys white blood cells, which are essential for fighting cancer when treatment is over. This weakening of the immune system can lead to a life-threatening condition called leukopenia, in which white blood cells drop to such low levels that they may be unable to fight off infections. When leukopenia sets in, treatment must be delayed in order to allow the white blood cell count to rise to a healthier level.

Here's the ideal chemotherapy scenario: white blood cells consistently stay at adequate levels so that treatment can proceed on schedule and the patient is not overly vulnerable to infection. Chlorella may measurably assist patients in achieving that goal. In Japan, chlorella extract is renowned for its ability to stimulate the immune system and support the growth of white blood cells at times of illness or treatments.

Higher White Blood Cell Counts Through Chlorella

Mice treated with the chemotherapy drug 5-fluorouracil (5FU) were given chlorella extract. Mice in the chlorella group showed faster recovery of white blood cells in bone marrow, maintained consistently higher levels of white blood cells throughout the study, and experienced complete recovery of white blood cells 20% faster than mice in the control group. [6] (figure 6)

Mice who were given a chlorella extract were administered the chemotherapy drug cyclophosphamide. These mice showed a white

Figure 6

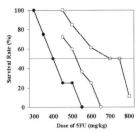

Effect of C. vulgaris glycoprotein (CVS) on LD50 of 5-fluorouracil (5FU). Mice were injected with CVS: 50 mg/kg (○) or 500 mg/kg (□) or none (●), and were treated with 5FU at the doses indicated. Survival was recorded daily for 20 days.

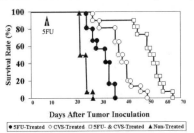

Effect of combination of CVS and 5FU on the survival in mice bearing MethA tumor.

● 5FU-Treated   ○ CVS-Treated   □ 5FU- & CVS-Treated   ▲ Non-Treated

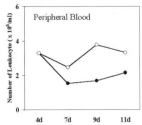

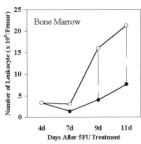

Effect of CVS on the number of leukocytes in peripheral blood (A) and bone marrow (B) of 5FU-treated mice. CDF1 mice were injected with CVS (50 mg/kg. six times, s.c.) on days - 14 to day - 1 and were treated with 5FU (250) mg/kg, i.p.) on day 0. ● 5FU-treated mice, ○ 5FU-and CVS-treated mice.

blood cell count that was 1.5 to 2 times higher than those in the control group. Both groups of mice were then injected with E. coli bacteria. Chlorella-treated mice had an astonishing 10 times more white blood cells at infection sites than the controls! The researchers termed this development "remarkable."[2]

Patients who are treated with immune-suppressing drugs sometimes develop a serious herpes-type virus called cytomegalovirus. Mice were given chlorella extract, then injected with lethal doses of this virus. Chlorella stimulated the activity of gamma interferon, an important immune system protein which helped launch an attack on the virus. Mice treated with chlorella survived the fatal virus and showed 35-42% decrease in virus replication. [3]

These studies indicate that chlorella can play an important role in activating the immune system during chemotherapy. But chlorella can do more: it can also help smooth the physical traumas of chemotherapy by reducing side-effects. Chemotherapy patients who take chlorella have noted they feel more energy and sleep sounder. Some people say their hair doesn't fall out as much and their skin doesn't feel as dry.

Minimizing Damage From Radiation

Like chemotherapy, radiation can devastate developing white blood cells. This assault on the immune system weakens patients and leaves them vulnerable to disease. But there is good news: studies show that chlorella can protect white cells from radiation destruction and enable them to recover faster.

● When mice were exposed to irradiation, they experienced a 25-40% reduction in the number of damaged bone marrow cells, if they were treated with chlorella. [45]

● Mice who were subjected to gamma-rays showed an "almost complete recovery" of colony forming units in the bone marrow, when they were given chlorella. Colony forming units are an early developmental stage of white blood cells, which eventually grow into a variety of immune cells. [46] (figure 7)

Researchers studying the effect of chlorella on radiation damage note that it is important to administer chlorella at exactly the right time. Chlorella should be given no earlier than one hour before radiation or no later than 15 minutes after radiation to be effective.

In addition, evidence suggests that people undergoing radiation treatment should take both chlorella tablets and chlorella extract. This combination ensures that patients receive the full range of immune-boosting nutrients during this crucial treatment period.

Fighting The Spread of Tumors

The goal of cancer therapy is to wipe out the disease at its source and prevent it from spreading. This goal is not always reachable. Sometimes surgery can contribute to the problem by opening a tumor, enabling the cancer cells to escape and spread. And sometimes the surgeon can not completely remove a tumor, because it's intertwined with vital

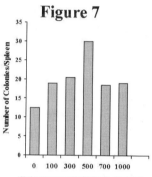

Figure 7

Effect of different concentrations of chlorella on the number of endogenous spleen colonies. Mice were fed 1 hr before irradiation with 8 Gy.

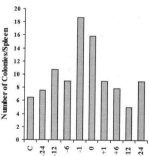

Effect of chlorella (500 mg/kg body wt.) fed orally at different time intervals before (-) or after (+) 8 gy whole body irradiation on the number of endogenous spleen colonies.

organs or tissues.

Because of these issues, chlorella's ability to fight tumors could be of paramount importance. Studies indicate that chlorella may be particularly adept at controlling the spread of tumors to other sites in the body, through its enhancement of immune system function.

- 50% of mice pre-treated with chlorella extract experienced complete disappearance of tumor mass. In the control group, the tumors progressively grew until death. The study showed that chlorella stimulated the performance of T-cells, which are important players in the immune system, sending them to infiltrate tumor sites. The researchers noted that pre-surgical treatment with chlorella extract may help prevent the spreading of tumors to other sites and inhibit tumor progression. [22]

- A Japanese study in *The Journal of Ethnopharmacology* reported that mice who were administered chlorella extract before they were injected with tumor cells, had a significant increase of survival times — as much as 300%. Control mice died within 20 days, while 73-80% of the chlorella-treated mice survived over 60 days. [47]

- Mice who were fed a daily diet of chlorella powder for 35 days before tumor inoculation and 22 days after showed a significant decrease (54% inhibition) of tumor growth. The study noted that chlorella increased immune system activity and lengthened the survival time of the tumor-bearing mice. [48]

A Fascinating Study: Cancer Patients and Chlorella

A 1990 clinical trial at The Medical College of Virginia examined the effect of chlorella supplements on 20 patients with brain tumors over a two-year period. In addition to receiving traditional treatments for brain tumors, such as radiation, chemotherapy and medications, these patients took approximately 100 chlorella tablets (20 grams) and five ounces of chlorella extract daily.

- 90% of patients maintained normal red blood cell levels, at the end of four months.

- 90% of patients showed normal white blood cell counts at the end of eight months.

- Patients complained of fewer colds and respiratory infections than expected, and reported that chlorella increased their strength.

- Among the patients who showed suppressed immune system response at the start of the study, five out of six achieved normal levels after four months.

In cases where the disease was advanced, chlorella did not stop its progression. But in less severe cases, especially in younger patients, chlorella seemed to increase the time before tumor recurrence and lengthen longevity. At the end of the two-year study, seven patients were still alive and showed no signs of tumor reappearance. [5]

Of course, these results need to be duplicated in large scale studies. But they do offer intriguing evidence of chlorella's ability to complement traditional cancer therapies with nutrients that boost and bolster the immune system.

What Cancer Patients Must Know About Taking Chlorella

The accumulated evidence suggests that cancer patients should keep in mind the following:

- Chlorella does not cure cancer. It should never be taken as a substitute for other forms of cancer treatment. Instead, it works best as a complement to conventional treatments, enhancing the immune system and improving quality of life.

- Patients at serious risk of infection or with a severely compromised immune system need to take significantly higher daily doses of chlorella than the normal recommended amount.

- To be most effective, chlorella should be taken before treatments that suppress the immune system or before exposure to infection. This gives the immune cells time to multiply and grow, so they can do their best work.

- Take chlorella in both tablet form and as a liquid extract. Both forms of chlorella contain nutrients that revitalize the immune system, but they are not identical. The liquid extract contains a concentration of some of the best immune supporters, but it does not contain all the elements found in the tablet. By taking both, you can be assured of maximum potency and a full range of nutrients.

Helping Cancer Patients Through Treatment And Beyond

Chlorella can help cancer patients throughout the ordeal of treatment and support them in their long-term struggle to maintain health. Cancer patients who take chlorella during treatment may experience higher white blood cell counts, fewer infections, increased strength and vitality and enhanced immune system function. And after chemotherapy and radiation have ended, those who continue to take chlorella may benefit from its power to energize the immune system and curtail the spread of tumors.

CHAPTER 16
The Mystery of Epstein-Barr

"I'm sorry, there's nothing I can do for you." How frustrating it is to hear your doctor say those words when you feel so sick. People who suffer from Epstein-Barr virus (EBV) find themselves trapped in a prison of exhaustion and pain, without any known treatment to free them.

95% Of The U.S. Population Has Epstein-Barr Virus

EBV is an astoundingly common virus - an incredible 95% of the US population has it! It's transmitted through infected saliva, usually during childhood, when children share toys they have put in their mouth, or during adolescence, through kissing.

In most people, the virus lies dormant and harmless for the rest of their life. But in a small percentage of people, it reactivates, causing serious, debilitating mononucleosis.

For people with EBV, holding down a job can be a challenge. They suffer from extreme fatigue, aching muscles, and flu-like symptoms that can make working impossible. Doctors can only offer symptomatic relief, since no anti-viral drugs are available.

"A Significant Improvement in Their Condition"

Yet doctors who prescribe chlorella to their patients with EBV are impressed by the results. Dr. David Steenblock, of the Health Restoration Medical Clinic in Mission Viejo, California, uses chlorella in his practice for a variety of ailments. Dr. Steenblock says, "It was through a special interest in the Epstein-Barr virus that I was able to observe personally the effectiveness of this food supplement. When it was administered to several patients diagnosed with EBV, there was a significant improvement in their condition."

One of Dr. Steenblock's patients, Marie Baer, is a teacher who was so exhausted from EBV that she arrived late for her classes and went to bed right after work. Weekends were spent sleeping, trying to regain energy. Under Dr. Steenblock's guidance, she improved her diet and began taking chlorella daily. She regained her energy and is, once again, able to carry her full work load.

"I Was Going To Quit My Job"

Neal Spearing is another patient of Dr. Steenblock's, who suffered from EBV. He was so exhausted that he was on the verge of quitting his job, when he came to Dr. Steenblock, who started him on a nutritional regimen that included chlorella. His stamina improved to the point where he could work full-time with enough energy to paint his garage on weekends.

A Clever Virus That Plays Hide and Seek

Epstein-Barr virus is particularly adept at tricking the immune system and shielding itself from attack. It knows how to raise a molecular flag that makes it appear to be part of your body's home team, instead of an enemy invader. With this clever camouflage, EBV hides in plain sight, staving off attack by immune system cells.

Scientists have much to learn about successfully foiling EBV and other viruses. But as they explore potential treatments, one fact remains indisputable: to fight off a virus, your immune system should function on the highest possible level.

Chlorella Pumps Up Your Immune System

Chlorella is a proven stimulator of the immune system. Numerous tests have documented its ability to increase the efficiency of your cell metabolism, support the production of interferon, a powerful natural antiviral agent, and elevate your white blood cell count.

To help prevent an attack of Epstein-Barr virus or to lessen its severity, add chlorella's immune-boosting nutrients to your daily self-care regimen.

CHAPTER 17
Chronic Fatigue Syndrome

Like so many ailments in which exhaustion is the main symptom, Chronic Fatigue Syndrome (CFS) was long considered a psychiatric problem. People who experienced prolonged fatigue, fever, and joint pain were diagnosed as depressed and treated as if their illness was imaginary.

Today, however, researchers have discovered specific biochemical symptoms that are associated with CFS, and it is recognized as a genuine illness. Although its cause remains elusive, researchers are honing in on what may trigger CFS and which approaches can offer maximal relief. And at the forefront of these new approaches is nutritional supplementation.

"When I Don't Take Chlorella, I'm Literally Exhausted"

Chlorella, with its wealth of health-building nutrients, can be a powerful addition to the diet of someone suffering from CFS. Linda Atchinson of Humbolt, Tennesse says, "I have been taking chlorella for over a year. I originally started taking it because I had chronic fatigue. It has helped this condition tremendously. I have so much more energy. I also think that chlorella has helped my immune system. I don't catch colds and viruses as often."

And Barbara Franklin of Chesapeake Beach, Maryland says, "I had chronic fatigue when I started taking chlorella. Yes, I can feel the difference. When I don't take it, I'm literally exhausted, but if I keep taking it, I feel pretty good."

Support Your Adrenal Gland with Chlorella

One of the leading theories about CFS is that it is caused by a malfunction of the hypothalamus, a pea-sized area of the brain which coordinates traffic between the brain and immune system. When something goes wrong with the hypothalamus, the adrenal glands grow sluggish, inviting in the flu-like symptoms of CFS. The authors of *The Brain Wellness Plan* advocate that people with CFS nutritionally support their adrenal glands with vitamin C, zinc and vitamin B-6. Chlorella contains all these nutrients.

Most patients with CFS show a weak immune system response. Therefore, if you suffer from CFS, you should supply your immune system with nutrients that are clinically-proven to support and stimulate it. Zinc, vitamin A, the full range of B vitamins, vitamin C and vitamin E are all good news for your immune system, and chlorella contains them all.

Another implicating factor in CFS is candida yeast overgrowth. These unfriendly bacteria can enjoy explosive population growth in your intestines, where they produce over 75 toxic substances. Their waste products interfere with your digestion and sap your strength. Here again, chlorella can support your recovery. Chlorella enhances the growth of "friendly" bacteria in your intestinal system, thereby helping to vanquish the poison-producing candida yeast.

Get Back On Your Feet and Enjoy Life Again

If you suffer from CFS, you need powerful nutritional support to rebuild your health. Chlorella can provide you with nutrients that stimulate your immune system, support your adrenal glands and restore good health to your digestive system. Collectively, these nutrients can go to work, dramatically restoring your vim and vigor, as they did for Richard Davis of Palos Verdes, California: "I was diagnosed with chronic fatigue syndrome 6/01/97. I started taking chlorella 7/01/97. Since then, my fatigue is 95% removed and I have not missed a day of work as a result of fatigue in over a year."

CHAPTER 18
Bowel Disorders

Chlorella has a unique ability to balance and normalize body functions, and nowhere do we see this power more strikingly than in the bowel. Dr. Randall E. Merchant, a researcher who uses chlorella in his clinical trials, finds that when he gives chlorella to patients with constipation, the constipation gets better. But when he gives chlorella to patients with diarrhea, the diarrhea gets better. Although this seems paradoxical, the reason is that in both instances, chlorella brings the body back into balance.

The All Too Common Problem of Constipation

As we grow older, many of us battle chronic constipation. Although it might seem like a minor annoyance, constipation is actually a serious threat to your health. Toxins linger in the bowel far too long, breeding disease in that area, and seeping poisons into the bloodstream. Every organ in the body can be dragged down by the bowel. Fatigue, headaches, bad breath and cancer of the colon and breast are all associated with constipation.

Chlorella provides significant relief to constipation sufferers. Japanese researchers have determined that chlorella increases peristalsis, the rhythmic contractions which force waste products onward. Other studies show that chlorella encourages the growth of friendly bacteria in the digestive system and discourages the growth of harmful ones.

In addition, chlorella's protein and nucleic acids can significantly repair damaged tissue and rebuild irritated bowel walls.

These therapeutic activities can result in swift, dramatic improvements. A study of nursing home residents found that chlorophyll offered reliable relief for constipation. Many people who use chlorella regularly report similar results: "I had problems with bowel movements. I was constipated. Since taking chlorella, I don't have this problem anymore. And overall I feel better," says Patsy Davidson of Beaverton, Oregon, while Phyllis Sealy of Bathurst, North Dakota remarks, "Before I used to be bothered with constipation. Now since I've been taking chlorella, I am regular."

The Nightmare of Inflammatory Bowel Disease

If chlorella succeeds in relieving constipation, it also helps people suffering from the nightmare of chronic diarrhea. Dr. Randall E. Merchant conducted a study of chlorella's effect on inflammatory bowel disease (IBD) which yielded highly encouraging results.

IBD affects over two million Americans, including an estimated 200,000 children. IBD inflames the lining of the digestive tract, causing severe bouts of diarrhea, painful cramps and bloody stools. People with IBD often lose their appetite and experience serious weight loss. In severe cases, IBD sufferers are unable to work or even leave home.

IBD comes in two forms: ulcerative colitis and Crohn's disease. Dr. Merchant studied patients with ulcerative colitis, who suffer from inflammation of the innermost lining of the colon and rectum. Over a two month period, patients were given chlorella on a daily basis. Every patient showed significant improvement in all four categories of evaluation: stool frequency, rectal bleeding, mucosal appearance and general health. Prior to taking chlorella, the patients' average Disease Activity Index, which measured their overall severity of symptoms, was 7.2. After taking chlorella, the average Disease Activity Index was 2.8. [33]

The Mayo Clinic notes that standard treatment for IBD may include fiber supplements to bulk up the stool, iron supplements to reduce anemia from chronic bleeding, and vitamin B-12 to promote digestion and assimilation of food. Chlorella contains all of these nutrients.

Does Your Hot Dog Contain E.Coli?

One of chlorella's most important functions is battling dangerous, or even deadly bacteria in your bowels. In 1999, 35 million pounds of ready-to-eat meats were recalled, after widespread contamination with Listeria monocytogene was discovered. Listeria, which killed 425 people in 1998, is a lethal bacteria that can invade ready-to-eat meats after they are processed.

A study of chlorella's influence on Listeria yielded fascinating results. After a control group of mice was infected with Listeria all the mice died. But an infected group given a chlorella extract had a 20% to 55% survival rate, depending on the dose. [24]

Chlorella also vanquished E. coli, another deadly bacteria. Mice with suppressed immune systems who were given chlorella extract succeeded in eliminating lethal doses of E. coli. But the mice who did not receive the chlorella extract died within 24 hours. [2]

Keep It Moving, Keep It Clean

Chlorella's unique combination of ingredients can powerfully help to restore good bowel health. By normalizing the body's functioning, chlorella can assist constipated people in speeding up bowel transit time and cleaning out toxins. For people with diarrhea and inflammatory bowel disease, chlorella can repair damaged tissues and improve overall symptoms. And it can fight deadly bacteria and encourage the growth of friendly flora that are vital to the digestive process. Chlorella, "the great normalizer," can work wonders in the bowels.

CHAPTER 19
Heavy Metal Poisoning and Environmental Hazards

Chlorella is unique in its ability to detoxify your body. Blessed with cell walls that bind to toxins and the highest concentration of chlorophyll of any organism, chlorella safely escorts poisons out of your system that might otherwise linger for decades.

In a world infested with pollution, pesticides, food additives, heavy metals, and toxic chemicals, chlorella allows you to continually purge these health-robbers from your system. Exposure to toxins can come on the job, through food, air and water, from your carpet, furniture, cookware, and dozens of other sources — even from the inside of your own mouth.

Let's take a closer look at how chlorella cleans and purifies poisons from your system.

Pass the Mercury, Please

Fish is good for you: that's what the nutritionists tell us. And many people have made a conscientious effort in recent years to cut back on red meat and eat fish instead.

While it's true that fish is a terrific source of protein and omega fatty acids, the unpleasant fact is that fish can also be a source of mercury, a toxic heavy metal.

The worst offenders tend to be swordfish, shark and large tuna used for steaks and sushi. But depending on its environment, any fish can be contaminated with mercury including fresh-water fish.

Once mercury invades your system, it doesn't want to leave. It burrows into your cells and tissues, eventually being released into your bloodstream, where it perpetually circulates, spreading trouble. Mercury attacks the nervous system, the kidneys and various other organs. A host of problems, including fatigue, constipation, memory loss and high blood pressure, have been associated with mercury contamination.

Inside your mouth is another surprising source of mercury: dental fillings. Approximately half the fillings in the United States contain mercury. Whether they pose a health problem remains controversial. The American Dental Association says mercury fillings are safe, but some studies conclude that mercury from dental fillings can find its way into the circulatory system and thereby cause trouble.

Because both sources of contamination are so common, chlorella's ability to detoxify mercury is precious. In fact, *The Dental Amalgam Mercury Syndrome* newsletter specifically recommends chlorella as a way to cleanse mercury from your body.[11] Studies note that chlorella's sticky cell walls adhere to heavy metal deposits, wrap them up and remove them. And its high concentration of chlorophyll, the most powerful detoxifier in nature, works hard to cleanse the blood of heavy metal contamination.

Aluminum, Lead, and Cadmium: A Trio of Health Spoilers

Your body has no use for aluminum. When you drink water that contains aluminum-filled waste product or a settling agent called "alum," your body does not thank you. It may already feel overwhelmed with aluminum from your toothpaste, cooking pots, aspirin, lipstick, beer, tea, baking powder, deodorant and other household sources.

In fact, aluminum is everywhere and that's not good news for your brain or kidneys. Aluminum has been found in high doses in the brain cells of Alzheimer's patients. While that connection has not been definitively proven, aluminum is strongly associated with memory loss and the deterioration of learning abilities and motor skills.

Lead and cadmium are other heavy metals that can wreak havoc with your health. One of the most common metals in manufacturing, lead can easily invade your tap water, air and dinner plates, and from there, assault your brain. Cadmium, an immune system wrecker, may be found in your carpet backing, drinking water, processed food, and in the worst offender of all — cigarette smoke.

By taking chlorella on a regular basis, you can benefit from its proven ability to safely remove these dangerous heavy metals. For instance, in a study of people suffering from cadmium poisoning, eight grams of chlorella were administered daily. After 12 days, patients showed three times more cadmium in their excretions. After 24 days, that number had grown to seven times more cadmium. [7] And in another cadmium study, chlorella- treated rats who were given cadmium did not absorb the cadmium into their body and did not show stunted growth, unlike the rats in the control group. [8]

Insecticide, Step Outside!

Heavy metals aren't the only toxic disrupters of your body. A constant barrage of poisons are out there, trying to get in. Pesticides and insecticides, for instance, may enter uninvited through your food, a frighteningly common occurrence.

Here again, chlorella can serve as your shield and protector. According to a clinical study, chlordecone, a highly toxic insecticide, is removed twice as fast from the body when chlorella is taken. Chlorella-treated rats were spared the constant re-circulation of chlordecone through their system and eliminated this toxin in half the time as rats in the control group. [14]

"This property of detoxifying hydrocarbon pesticides and insecticides is very important in our world of constant chemical exposure and is one of the important differences between chlorella and other 'green' products," writes Dr. David Steenblock in *Chlorella, Natural Medicinal Algae*.

Purify Your Body Of Toxins

In a toxic world, chlorella is a remarkable gift. Safely, gently and naturally, it can remove dangerous chemicals from your body, protecting your health from the ravages of prolonged exposure to poison. With its sticky cell wall that binds up toxins and its high concentration of the legendary purifying agent, chlorophyll, this tiny green algae is a mighty warrior for good health and clean living.

CHAPTER 20
Healing Ulcers, Wounds and Sores

Diabetes and Foot Ulcers

Joseph never felt any pain in his foot, and that was the problem. As a diabetic, Joseph had lost all sensation in his lower limbs. He did not notice the open sore growing on the bottom of his foot until severe infection set in. By that time, it was too late for treatment, and his foot had to be amputated.

Joseph's story is all too common. Many diabetics suffer from foot ulcers which they fail to notice. Caused by narrowed arteries which reduce blood flow to the region, diabetic foot ulcers can fester and grow hopelessly infected.

Other Causes of Foot Ulcers

Although diabetes is the most common cause of foot ulcers, it is not the only one. High blood pressure and hardening of the arteries can disrupt circulation in the foot area, creating ripe condition for ulcers. And alcoholism, rheumatoid arthritis and systemic lupus can also be factors.

"Trauma — including burns, wounds and broken bones — are other big causes of foot ulcers," says Dr. Thom W. Rooke, a specialist in vascular disease at the Mayo Clinic in Minnesota. "When you bang your foot or your leg, you can trigger the beginning of an ulcer. In the United States, bed sores are also one of the most common causes of ulcers, and they may involve the foot."

Soothing Chlorella, Healer of Ulcers

If you suffer from an ulcer on your foot or elsewhere, you should seek medical attention immediately. You should also be aware of the healing power of chlorella. Chlorella contains more chlorophyll than any known plant, and for more than seventy years, chlorophyll has been recognized as a spectacular healer of wounds.

In 1943, doctors at the New York Post-Graduate Medical School determined that chlorophyll in ointment form successfully treated 19 out of 25 types of skin ulcers. The doctors noted that chlorophyll had a "stimulating effect" on the supportive tissues, promoting their rapid healing. [49]

In a major study of 1,372 experimentally induced wounds and burns, chlorophyll preparations were the only type to consistently promote healing. In fact, wound healing was accelerated by 24% and occurred in 67% of the cases. [50]

In a 1945 study, chlorophyll was used to treat infected ulcers. When used in combination with penicillin, the healing rate of wounds was accelerated by 35% over the use of either penicillin or chlorophyll by itself. [29]

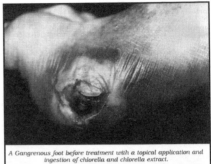

A Gangrenous foot before treatment with a topical application and ingestion of chlorella and chlorella extract.

Apply CGF, Watch What Happens

Some doctors, such as Dr. David Steenblock, use CGF, a liquid extract of chlorella, which they directly apply to the ulcer. "CGF in honey can be applied directly to the ulcer in generous amounts and held in place by the use of a non-sticking type of dressing over which are applied 4 x 4 gauze pads soaked in the

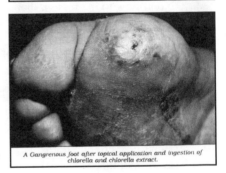

A Gangrenous foot after topical application and ingestion of chlorella and chlorella extract.

CGF. The purpose is to keep the ulcer saturated at all times with the CGF in honey. The person should keep entirely off their foot until healing is complete. A successful outcome is possible if the person carefully follows their physician's directions."

Because diabetic ulcers are so difficult to heal, it is vital that anyone with this condition be under a doctor's care. Foot ulcers can rapidly grow infected to the point where amputation is required. But some healing may be possible when a liquid extract of chlorella is topically applied, especially in combination with a rigorous course of antibiotics.

Internal Ulcers Respond To Chlorella Too

Chlorella not only heals skin ulcers, it heals internal ulcers, too. In Japan, patients with stomach and duodenal ulcers who were not responding to the usual medications were given chlorella. In most cases, the pain vanished within ten days of taking three grams daily of chlorella. Within 21 to 40 days, virtually all of the other symptoms disappeared. X-rays showed the ulcers had completely healed in the majority of patients, and a miniature medical camera proved that new tissue had closed up the ulcers. [30]

Dr. David Steenblock notes that a liquid extract of chlorella often provides immediate relief in problems of the upper intestinal tract, such as an irritated esophagus or stomach ulcer. Dr. Steenblock attributes this healing to the soothing effect of the chlorella liquid upon the internal tissues.

Why does chlorella have such a healing effect on ulcers and wounds? Perhaps the answer can be found in a landmark scientific study by Dr. Smith. He discovered that chlorophyll, when added to tissue culture, caused "an almost immediate growth response" of fibroblasts. Fibroblasts are the cells that the body uses to repair wounds. [28]

Diabetics: Be Vigilant, Be Knowledgeable

If you have diabetes, you need to be vigilant about monitoring your feet for signs of ulcers. You also need to know that chlorella can help with difficult-to-heal wounds. Chlorella can stimulate the body's own healing mechanism and provide dramatic relief for both external and internal wounds and ulcers.

CHAPTER 21
Protecting Your Eyesight

In a recent poll, people were asked their greatest fear. One out of four responded with "loss of vision." Our eyesight connects us with the world; yet, for too many people, blindness has been an inevitable part of growing older.

But if you take some simple health-building measures, you can protect and preserve your vision. Glaucoma, cataracts, diabetes and macular degeneration are conditions that develop gradually. You can stop them from beginning or progressing by adding specific nutritional supplements to your diet. In some cases, you can even reverse the deterioration of an eye disease and restore lost sight.

The Eyes Have It: Nutrients for Vision

In *The Eye Care Revolution*, Dr. Robert Abel, Jr. explains which nutrients have been clinically documented to support vision.

● **The carotenoids** (carotenes), which are related to vitamin A, are powerful antioxidants, protecting your eyes from the vicious damage of free radicals. Each carotenoid has a specific function within your optical system. Lutein, for instance, is a pigment in the center of the retina that shields you from ultraviolet light. Chlorella brims with carotenes, and is such a rich source of lutein that manufacturers are studying how to extract its lutein for medicinal purposes.

● **The B vitamins** work together as a group for proper nerve functioning within the eyes and body. Chlorella contains all the B vitamins.

● **Magnesium, iron, zinc** and **copper** are all minerals essential to your overall health and the functioning of your optical system. Magnesium improves vision in people with glaucoma and is associated with healthier eyes in diabetics. Zinc can play a role in stopping the progress of macular degeneration. Insufficient levels of zinc are known to cause vision problems. Every one of these important minerals can be found in chlorella.

● **Amino acids** are used by the body to create proteins. Chlorella contains all the essential amino acids. It is an excellent source of methionine, an amino acid which the body uses to manufacture taurine. Highly concentrated in the retina, taurine is associated with good vision and protection from macular degeneration.

Is Macular Degeneration A Hopeless Disease?

The leading cause of blindness in people over 65 is macular

degeneration. Caused by a deterioration of the center of the retina, it leads to a gradual loss of sight that can eventually rob you of the ability to read, drive or even distinguish faces.

Current mainstream medicine contends that nothing can be done to stop this devastating disease. But a new nutrition-based approach to treating macular degeneration suggests that, in fact, there are ways to not only arrest its progress, but even reverse it.

In January 1997, Dr. Charles Krall published an article in the *Townsend Letter for Doctors & Patients*, in which he described an experimental program of nutritional supplementation. Dr. Krall gave 41 antioxidants, minerals, and herbs to patients with macular degeneration. Six out of ten patients experienced improved vision. "This study supports the potential efficacy of a nutritional program to retard the usual deterioration that occurs with macular degeneration," wrote Dr. Krall. [51]

Chlorella Contains Nutrients That Fight Macular Degeneration

In *The Eye Care Revolution*, Dr. Abel strongly advocates treating macular degeneration with nutritional supplements. "Quite simply, the macula, the central portion of the retina, is very responsive to free-radical-fighting antioxidant nutrients…A study performed at the National Eye Institute (part of the National Institutes of Health) showed that, in many cases, diet and supplementation can delay or even stop vision loss due to macular degeneration," wrote Dr. Abel.

Dr. Abel recommends that people battling macular degeneration supplement their diet with carotenes (particularly lutein), zinc, essential fatty acids, and magnesium. Chlorella is an excellent source of all these nutrients.

Because macular degeneration is associated with poor digestion, Dr. Abel suggests that you try to improve the working of your digestive system. Chlorella encourages the growth of "friendly" bacteria in your intestines, which substantially aid in digestion. It also contains dietary fibers, which are crucial in keeping your bowels in top working order. By taking nutrients that improve your digestive functioning, you can help fight off macular degeneration. In the words of Dr. Abel, "What's good for the digestion is good for the macula."

Have The Foresight To Protect Your Vision

Chlorella brims with nutrients that nourish and shield your optical system. By taking chlorella on a regular basis, you have the foresight to protect your eyes and enjoy a long lifetime of acute vision.

CHAPTER 22
Preventing Memory Loss and Easing Stress

W here did I put my wallet? What was that phone number? Where did I park the car? The dreaded "brain fog" that descends on many older people seems an inevitable part of aging, and a possible frightening forecast of Alzheimer's and other forms of dementia. Studies have clearly established that free radicals, the rampaging molecules that attack your cellular structure, are major culprits in causing this mental decay, "rusting" your brain in the same oxidizing process that rusts metal.

But there's no need to let your brain rust away, when you can protect and revitalize it. Chlorella contains a host of antioxidants that defeat free radicals, thereby safeguarding your mental powers. Let's look at some intriguing ways that chlorella invigorates your brain and protects your memory from the nasty damage of free radicals.

Make Your Brain Happy: Give It Oxygen

Your brain needs oxygen and plenty of it. That is one reason why free radicals are so dangerous to your memory and other mental powers: they can reduce the oxygen supply to your brain. Here's how this unhealthy process works: free radicals encourage cholesterol to stick to your artery walls, creating narrow, inflexible blood passageways that reduce the flow of blood to your brain and elsewhere.

Chlorella can help prevent this process by lowering cholesterol levels and keeping artery walls flexible. Japanese patients who took chlorella daily for a year showed significantly lower cholesterol levels. [32] Rabbits who had chlorella added to their high-cholesterol diet displayed lower cholesterol levels than rabbits given the cholesterol-lowering drug Clofibrate. [34] And half the patients who took a small dose of chlorella for two months showed improved flexibility of their blood vessels. [35]

By keeping your blood flowing smoothly through your arteries, you enable your brain to stay active and alive.

Protect the Fuel Stations of Your Brain

Inside every cell in your brain is a "fuel station" which converts nutrients into energy. These mitochondria, as they are called, manufacture the mental energy you need to learn new information, store data and recall facts. Unfortunately, mitochondria are particularly vulnerable to attack by free radicals.

When the mitochondria in your brain are damaged, your brain literally runs out of energy. Your mental processes sputter and slow down and your memory suffers. However, clinical evidence now shows that chlorophyll has powerful antioxidant properties that protect your mitochondria from free radical assault.

In a study published in 2000, researchers documented their use of chlorophyll in protecting the mitochondria of mice. "Our results show that chlorophyll is highly effective in protecting mitochondria, even at a low concentration…," the authors of the study concluded. "When chlorophyll was fed to mice at a dose of 1% in drinking water, there was a significant reduction in the potential for oxidative damage in cell suspensions from liver, brain and testis."[52] Chlorella boasts a higher concentration of chlorophyll than any known substance, providing you with a simple, effective way to nourish your body with this brain protector.

A Landmark 20 Year Study Says: Eat Your Beta-Carotene!

In a 1997 article entitled "The Relation Between Antioxidants and Memory Performance in the Old and Very Old", researchers detailed the results of a study that spanned 20 years. People who regularly consumed high levels of the antioxidants beta-carotene and vitamin C performed notably better on memory tests. In particular, they showed greater ability to learn and retain facts. [53]

That's good news for chlorella users, because chlorella is a superb source of beta-carotene. In fact, it contains six times more beta-carotene than that famous green health-builder, spinach! Chlorella also contains a wealth of other antioxidants which effectively disarm free radicals and shield your mental acuity.

Don't Let A Bull Loose In The China Shop Of Your Brain

We get antioxidants in two ways: we eat them and we manufacture them in our body. The antioxidants that we manufacture from protein enzymes are extraordinarily potent. Of all of these, SOD (superoxide dismutase enzyme) is one of the most crucial for brain function.

SOD has the all-important task of cleaning up a vicious free radical in the brain. "If that SOD enzyme is ineffective in clearing the brain of that toxic free radical, however, the destructive effect to healthy cells is equivalent to turning a herd of bulls loose in a china shop, with free radicals causing rampant destruction," writes Dr. Jay Lombard and Carl Germano in *The Brain Wellness Plan*. Reduced levels of SOD have been associated with serious brain disorders, including amyotrophic lateral sclerosis (Lou Gehrig's Disease).

Given how vital the manufacture of SOD is for your mental powers, it is interesting to note that mice who were given chlorella extract generated levels of SOD that were $1^1/2$ times higher than those of mice in the control group. [54]

Stress And Your Brain: How to Fight Back

At times of great stress, you may feel as if you're "losing your mind." You may feel so burned out and weighed down with worry that you have trouble concentrating and remembering necessary information. The truth is: you're right. You are losing brain cells.

Emotional stress bombards your brain with hormones that damage your ability to learn and memorize. Over prolonged periods, this damage can be serious, interfering with your ability to regenerate brain cells that control memory and learning.

Chlorella gently protects the brain from the destructive hormones unleashed by stress. Over a 14-day period, mice were exposed to severe psychological stress. The mice who were given chlorella extract showed "significantly suppressed" levels of stress hormones. Despite their intense environmental challenges, these mice were able to maintain relatively normal levels of stress hormones. [55]

"Chlorella Has Changed My Outlook to One of Optimism"

What's good for mice is good for you. One of the most pleasant and perhaps unexpected byproducts of taking chlorella is that it encourages a feeling of inner happiness and serenity that can withstand a surprising amount of brutal everyday stress and strain.

Brenda Laney of Wickenburg, Arizona writes, "I work as a 911 operator and a police, fire and ambulance dispatcher. As a communications officer, I struggle through shift changes and endure stress on a daily basis... Before taking the chlorella, I had a problem with eating healthy, sleeping and discomfort due to stomach aches and nerves from stress. After being on the chlorella for three to four weeks, I noticed a drastic change in my eating habits; I was losing weight and I also had an increase in energy...I feel very good and will never stop taking chlorella!"

Lorraine Andrade of Montebello, California says, "After taking chlorella I find my health is in stronger physical and mental form, and my mood to be more stable...My energy level is higher and I feel more alert. Overall, chlorella is an excellent balancer and cleanser for the body and mind."

R.S. Blake of Palm Bay, Florida says, "Chlorella has definitely changed my outlook to one of optimism. I have a great deal more energy and feeling of well-being."

Thanks for the Memories, Chlorella!

Behind these emotional feelings are biochemical facts. Because the nutrients in chlorella suppress the hormones created by stress, you can remain calm and in control, even during a busy, turbulent day. Not only do you appreciate life more, but you protect your brain from the long-term damage of stress hormones.

When you take chlorella, you are protecting your brain from the constant toll of stress and the frightening damage of free radicals. And even better, you are fueling your brain to achieve a long life of acute mental powers, of learning that never ends and memory that never fades.

CHAPTER 23
Malnutrition and Aging

"I just don't feel like eating." Many older people utter these words with alarming frequency, no matter how tempting the meal placed before them. As their food intake declines, their strength deteriorates and they grow more vulnerable to disease.

Malnutrition is a serious problem among the elderly, affecting one out of four. As we age, our sense of taste and smell can radically diminish. With dulled taste buds on the tongue and inactive nerves in the nose, food seems bland and unappealing. Medication can compound the problem, often making food taste bitter.

The Challenge of Three Square Meals A Day

There are other reasons that older people don't eat enough. Sometimes chewing is difficult, because of missing teeth or ill-fitting dentures. Constipation and other digestive problems are all too common in this age group, further discouraging appetite.

Even for seniors who love to eat, consuming three solid meals a day can be difficult. Going to the supermarket, carrying heavy bags of groceries, cooking a meal and cleaning up afterwards demand strength and stamina that is beyond the capabilities of many older people.

Some recent studies indicate the breadth of the problem. A survey of elderly people who considered themselves "health-conscious" was conducted in Albuquerque, New Mexico. Eighty-six percent of the women and 85% of the men lacked the minimum recommended amounts of vitamins B-6, B-12, E and D, folic acid, calcium and zinc.

For people in a nursing home where food options are limited, the problem of getting adequate nutrition can be particularly acute. Institutional meals can be unappetizing, and all too frequently, their nutritional content is woefully inadequate. A startling study of 14 nursing homes revealed that not one of them met the recommended daily amounts for all nutrients in the food they served their patients.

More Years, Less Absorption of Nutrients

The result of constant under-nourishment can be a serious erosion of health. When you lack proper nutrition day after day, your body weakens. You grow tired, listless and fragile. Chronic ailments take root and serious disease can flourish. The situation becomes a vicious circle, in which the weaker you grow, the less you eat and the more malnourished you become.

Even the food you do eat is probably not adequately absorbed. As the body ages, its ability to utilize nutrients declines. Many older people lack a healthy amount of digestive enzymes, which leads to trouble in breaking down and absorbing nutrients. Vitamin B-12, in particular, is a crucial nutrient that is notoriously difficult for older people to handle.

And, of course, many elders retain bad eating habits they have acquired over a lifetime. According to a United States Senate report, the average American consumes a diet that is mostly empty of nutritional content, with 40% of its calories as fat and 20% as refined sugar. Sadly, fewer than 30% of Americans eat the recommended five daily servings of fruits and vegetables.

Chlorella Is The Perfect Supplement For Your Golden Years

For all of these reasons, supplementing your diet with chlorella makes sense as you grow older. Let's take a closer look at what chlorella can do for you in your senior years:

- Provide you with crucial nutrients that are often deficient in people over 60, including vitamins B-6, B-12, E, folic acid and zinc.
- Stimulate your digestive system to ease constipation and other stomach problems, thereby increasing appetite.
- Increase the efficiency of your cell metabolism, allowing for greater absorption of nutrients.
- Offer a simple way to take in a broad spectrum of nutrients, even if your appetite is low.
- Offset the decline of RNA production in your body by providing a rich whole-food source of nucleic acids.
- Stimulate the body's declining ability to manufacture antioxidants, thereby protecting your cells from free radical damage.
- Provide a host of nutrients you cannot find in pills, including a full range of carotenoids. Most vitamins only contain one of them, beta-carotene.

Bowling and Golfing at 84

Many older people who use chlorella believe that its nutrients give them youthful energy and reliable good health. They feel the keen difference when their bodies are fully nourished.

Kathryne Labonte of Kaneohe, Hawaii: "I am very pleased with chlorella, and am 79 going on 80...My work day begins at 4:30 A.M. to whenever I finish, which for 20 years has been 12 hours a day."

And Frederick Rouse of San Francisco, California: "I am 84 years old. I used to get colds one after another and the flu three or four times a year. Since I have been using chlorella, I haven't had a cold. I bowl twice a week and golf once and have more energy than before. I will continue chlorella as long as I live."

Full Nourishment for Glowing Health

Chlorella is a perfect choice to help ensure your body is wholly nourished, so you can enjoy your golden years in glowing health. With a full spectrum of nutrients to support your system, you can continue to enjoy the vitality of youth, decade after decade.

CHAPTER 24

Chlorella For The Whole Family: Children, Adults, Seniors And Pets

E very member of the family can enjoy chlorella. From the youngest child to the most venerable great-grandparent, chlorella can provide superb natural nutrition, perfectly targeted for each stage of life. Even the family pet can benefit from chlorella's steadfast, health-building gifts.

Chlorella for Children:

As a parent, you worry about your child receiving the right nutrition. You want to do everything you can to make sure your child grows up healthy and strong. That's why you should know about the positive effects chlorella can have on your child's development.

First of all, chlorella can provide your child with crucial nutritional support for growth. A Japanese study examined the effect of chlorella on the growth rate of ten-year-old fifth graders. Twenty-two boys and eighteen girls were given two grams of chlorella per day for 112 days. Boys grew an average of one inch; boys in the control group who did not take chlorella grew 0.6 inch. The average weight gain of the boys who took chlorella was 2.3 pounds; boys in the control group only gained 1.6 pounds. As for the girls, both groups grew 0.9 inch in height. But the girls who took chlorella gained an average of 4.2 pounds, while the control group gained 2.7 pounds. [56]

Protecting Your Child From Toxic Assault

Furthermore, in a world of environmental toxins, chlorella can help protect your child. The Federal Drug Administration finds pesticide residue in 30 - 40% of the food it samples. Inevitably, your child is eating food contaminated with toxic chemicals. To make matters worse, your child is breathing air clogged with pollutants, and drinking water that probably contains a host of undesirable chemicals.

Children's bodies are vulnerable to toxic assault. The overwhelming number of children suffering from asthma may reflect the ever-higher levels of pollutants and toxins to which they are exposed. You can help purify your child's system with chlorella, whose ability to safely remove toxins from the body is documented by reams of scientific evidence.

Does Your Child Eat Junk Food?

An unfortunate fact of American life is that children eat too much junk food. A gigantic marketing complex exists to cleverly ply them with sugar-filled cereal, candy and snacks. Even if you are strict about their diet, they will eat junk food at school and in their friends' homes. Not only is junk food filled with chemical additives, it disrupts their entire system and spoils their appetite for healthy food.

By giving your child chlorella, you provide a daily supply of crucial nutrients for their health, no matter how lamentable the rest of their diet may be. Every day, your child will receive a broad spectrum of vitamins, minerals, amino acids, nucleic acids and other nutrients that strongly support and protect his or her precious health.

Is Your Child A Prime Candidate for Chlorella?

Certain children are particularly in need of chlorella's nourishing powers. According to a study conducted at Nagasaki University in Japan, children in the following groups are primary candidates for chlorella:

- Children who exhibit poor growth
- Children who frequently suffer from colds, flu and fever
- Children with asthma
- Children with frequent dermatitis
- Children with frequent diarrhea and bloody stool
- Children with poor complexions

How To Give Your Child Chlorella

If you are an expectant mother, you can take chlorella as a daily supplement to pass on to your growing baby. It is recommended, however, that you consult with your physician about taking chlorella while you are pregnant. Once your baby is born, she can receive chlorella through your breast milk, if you take the supplements.

As your baby starts solid food, you can mix tablets or granules in with his or her food. Chlorella's mild flavor allows you to inconspicuously add it to soups, vegetable and fruit purees and even flour for bread. And you can easily add the liquid extract to vegetable juices.

The general rule is to give your child one tablet (200 mg) per year in age. So when your nine-year-old son finally figures out how to swallow pills, give him nine little green tablets (1800 mg). Tablets can be crushed and added to soft foods such as applesauce.

Chlorella For Adults:

The adult years are a time of enormous stress. You may be working long hours at your job, raising a family and perhaps caring for older parents, all at the same time. The pressures are unrelenting, and with so many responsibilities, you can't afford to get sick.

That's why it's supremely important to take care of yourself during these high-pressured years. Unfortunately, with all the demands on our day, many of us neglect our health. Without enough time to prepare nutritious meals, we tend to snack on junk food and eat highly-processed products rife with chemical additives. We don't exercise regularly or practice stress control techniques.

Worn Out, Burned Out And Down In The Dumps

The result is that an overwhelming number of adults feel exhausted, burned out and depressed. Insomnia is rampant and so are aches, pains and other chronic complaints. We desperately need our health, yet we never quite feel healthy enough.

During these all-important years when you need your energy most, chlorella can positively transform your health. Its remarkable nutrients can infuse you with energy and stamina that you haven't felt for years, brighten your mood and gently ease your anxieties. Chlorella can sharpen your mental powers, help you sleep nights, boost your sexual drive and relieve a host of physical vexations. In short, chlorella can help you cope with the endless demands of your life.

Furthermore, chlorella can stave off serious illnesses that are trying to mount a secret attack. Somewhere in your body there may be vulnerable points where disease-causing agents are burrowing in to wreak havoc over the long haul. Life-threatening illnesses like cancer and heart disease or painful ailments like arthritis and fibromyalgia can silently arrive, biding their time for months or even years till, suddenly, they announce themselves with a major health crisis. Chlorella can help your body fight off these happiness wreckers and safeguard your health for your golden years.

Are You A Prime Candidate For Chlorella?

While all adults can benefit from chlorella, some people may particularly profit from its nutritional riches. Dr. Michael Rosenbaum notes the following groups of prime candidates:

- People who suffer from fatigue and low stamina.
- People with fertility problems.
- Women with severe menopausal disorders.
- People who want greater sex drives.
- People with poor complexion or frequent dermatitis.
- People who experience hair loss.
- People with hypertension, constipation, stiffness of the shoulders, palpitation, headache, nervousness, dizziness, cold hands and cold feet, etc.
- Diabetes patients who also have hypertension.
- People with weak liver functioning whose blood needs to be cleaned.

Chlorella for Seniors:

The senior years should be a time of relaxation and enjoyment. After a lifetime of hard work, you should be able to spend time with friends and family, explore new interests and volunteer in your community. But for all too many people, serious health problems rob these years of their potential pleasure.

Chronic pain hobbles many seniors and low energy sidelines them at home. Those who are on medication often suffer from unpleasant, debilitating side effects. Compounding these problems, cellular efficiency decreases as we age and so does our ability to absorb nutrients.

Feel Young Again

For all these reasons, chlorella is an ideal supplement for seniors seeking to improve their health and recover their youthful vigor. Chlorella:

- promotes a high-functioning immune system so you can ward off disease.
- restores bowel regularity.
- improves cellular efficiency.
- sharpens memory and increases mental alertness and concentration.
- promotes healthy blood pressure levels.
- boosts energy and elevates mood.
- rebuilds damaged tissue.
- gives new hope to people with chronic diseases.

Are You On Medication? Here's What You Should Know

An important fact to note: Because chlorella is a natural whole food, it should not interfere with your medication. In fact, in the best case scenario, chlorella will enable you to lessen your dependence on medication (under the supervision of your doctor, of course) by allowing your body to naturally heal itself.

Chlorella For Pets:

People who discover the joy of chlorella often want to share it with their pets — and with good reason. The same nutritional banquet that transforms your health can powerfully work on your cat and dog, too (and your bird, hamster, rabbit and mouse).

In fact, pet owners are often stunned by the positive changes they see when their animal begins regularly taking chlorella. Fur or feathers grows shinier, energy levels rocket, allergies decrease and the overall health of their pet improves.

Why Your Pet Needs Chlorella

The truth is that your pet might be the family member most in need of chlorella's detoxifying powers. Pets are frequently exposed to poisons. Dogs that frolic on the grass can pick up dangerous residues of lawn and garden treatments, which they ingest when they lick their fur. And pets treated for fleas and ticks may become beautifully pest-free — but full of harmful chemicals.

These toxins can linger in fat cells for years, eventually attacking your pet's nerves, hormones and immune system. By providing your pets with daily servings of chlorella, you purify toxins from their system and protect their long-term health.

Healthy Chow for A Healthy Pet

What exactly is in the food you serve your pet? The answer could be downright unsavory. Horror stories abound of diseased animal flesh and contaminated grains. In 1999, 25 dogs died from eating chow infested with aflatoxin, a mold that develops in improperly stored grains. Several national recalls of dry pet foods have also highlighted the aflatoxin problem.

When you feed your pets chlorella, you provide them with high-quality food manufactured under scrupulously sanitary conditions. You supplement the often mediocre nutritional content of their food with superb ingredients that reinvigorate their health. And you protect them from possible contaminants in their chow by cleansing and purifying their system.

Chlorella is available in forms designed to be tasty and appealing to your pet.

The Family Friend: Chlorella Through The Ages

"Chlorella provides nutritional support for every stage of our lives," writes Dr. David Steenblock. "In youth, chlorella provides the building blocks necessary for growth. In adulthood, it provides nutrition to maintain optimal health and performance. And as we age, cell vitality is lost, and it becomes increasingly difficult to absorb the nutrients necessary to invigorate and restore cells... As President of the Aging Research Institute, I have conducted research on numerous food supplements and find chlorella to be an essential addition to any 'anti-aging' diet."

CHAPTER 25
How To Choose and Use Chlorella

Not all chlorella is created equal. In fact, some brands are vastly superior to others. So how do you choose which brand will provide you with the highest quality product?

To find the answer, let's take a close look at chlorella's cell wall. This unique substance is one of the supreme glories of chlorella. Its stickiness allows it to bind with heavy metals, pesticides and toxins such as P.C.B.s and safely carry them out of the body. And its extraordinary toughness provides such impenetrable protection that chlorella has flourished for 2.5 billion years, making it the oldest organism on earth.

Which Brand Is Best?

But while the unbreakable toughness of its cell wall is good for chlorella, it's bad for your digestion. Your body simply cannot digest chlorella with its cell wall intact. In order for you to smoothly absorb chlorella and gain full access to its interior nutrients, you must take chlorella whose cell walls have been broken down.

Therefore, one sure-fire way to discern a brand's quality is to learn which process is used to break down the cell wall. Inferior brands use heat or chemicals, which are largely ineffective in breaking down the wall. Furthermore, they have the unfortunate side effect of destroying much of the cell's nutritional value. The superior brand uses a completely mechanical method which was patented under the name DYNO-Mill™. Invented by Hideo Nakayama, this process thoroughly pulverizes the cell wall while preserving the integrity of the nutrients inside.

Dr. David Steenblock, author of *Chlorella, Natural Medicinal Algae*, notes the following difference in total digestibility of the chlorella cell:

DYNO-Mill™-processed cells..................**79%**

Heated and blanched cells....................**50%**

"Intact" cells **47%**

The superiority of the DYNO-Mill™ method was borne out by a study with young animals. Those who were fed DYNO-Mill™-processed chlorella had a 47% weight gain after 22 days. Animals fed the heat-treated chlorella showed a 39% weight gain, and animals fed no chlorella gained a mere 22%.

Five Hallmarks of A Superior Brand

According to a noteworthy report by The Japan Chlorella Treatment Association, "the chlorella tablets on the market are of widely varying quality." The Association urged caution in choosing a brand and listed five requirements of a superior chlorella product.

Microscopic Photography

Photo #1: Commonly available chlorella claiming to have a broken cell wall, which may not be easily digested or assimilated, losing nutritional value.

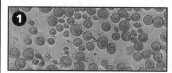

Photo #2: True broken cell chlorella (Dyno-Mill patented process) which means optimum digestion and assimilation of chlorella's nutritional value into your body.

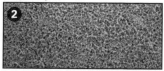

- The chlorella should be grown using a sanitary culturing method.

- It should contain a large protein content. Chlorella harvested in a centrifuge has significantly higher protein content. The Association noted "this is the kind of product to buy."

- The chlorella should be easily digestible.

- The tablet must disintegrate easily.

- The product should contain a large amount of Chlorella Growth Factor (CGF). Chlorella grown in dark places or indoors shows small CGF content, compared to chlorella that has multiplied in sunlight. The Association said, "It follows that unless one takes chlorella that has been cultured in sunlight, one cannot expect the product's outstanding results."

Smart Questions from A Savvy Consumer

Guided by these requirements, a consumer can ask the following questions to ensure their brand meets the highest possible standards:

- Do any certified independent laboratories test your product for contaminants?

- What process do you use to break down the cell walls?

- How often do you test your product internally?

- In what part of the world is your product grown?

● Is it grown in outdoor culture pools or closed indoor tanks?

If all this sounds overly complicated, relax. Choosing a brand is actually quite straightforward. Look for a brand that breaks down the cell wall with the DYNO-Mill™ method, grows its cells in outdoor fresh mineral water pools in areas of maximum sunlight and performs constant, rigorous testing. Then you can be confident your chlorella is of impeccable quality and meets the highest international standards.

How Do You Take Chlorella? A User's Guide

Now you have chosen your brand of chlorella. You are eager to begin enjoying its phenomenal health-giving powers. So how do you start?

In a word, gradually. Chlorella comes in tablets, granules and liquid extract. Most people begin with five tablets per day, or one gram of the granules, usually taken at meal time. If you are not used to eating fresh, raw vegetables, you may want to start with a smaller amount, such as one tablet per day.

Give your body a week or so to adjust to this new nutrient source. Then add another five tablets. After a week, add another five tablets, to reach a total of fifteen.

For the average adult, 15 tablets daily, or 3 grams of the granules, is the suggested amount. But you can safely add significant portions of chlorella to this baseline number if your health needs warrant it.

For instance, if you feel a cold or other illness coming on, take more chlorella. If you feel rundown and sluggish, take more chlorella. You can safely increase your servings above and beyond the recommended amount.

If you have a serious chronic illness, you should definitely consider establishing a higher daily baseline. "Many people with chronic viral conditions, such as Epstein-Barr virus or herpes virus, have shown significant improvements in their condition with larger amounts of chlorella. It is not unusual to find people who take 30-60 tablets daily (6-12 grams)," says Dr. David Steenblock.

You may also want to take a higher daily serving if you have a worrisome family medical history. "For example, if someone comes from a family history of cancer and both parents had cancer, then this person may want to take a fairly high dosage of chlorella because of the beta-carotene and other anti-cancer agents present," notes Dr. Steenblock.

For children, the rule of thumb is to give them one tablet per year of age. Therefore, a five-year-old child should take five tablets daily, and a ten-year-old should take ten.

Boost Your Immunity with Liquid Extract

Chlorella is also available as a liquid extract of concentrated CGF (Chlorella Growth Factor). CGF contains all the health-boosting nutrients found in the cell nucleus, including nucleic acids, peptides, and proteins.

Because CGF is associated with extraordinary immune-boosting powers, you should consider taking the liquid extract along with your tablets. This liquid extract is particularly important for older people, who can benefit from its powerful, easily-absorbed nutrients, and for people with chronic health problems.

Every tablet of chlorella contains CGF. But by supplementing the tablets with the liquid extract, you can intensify the healing power of CGF and enjoyed a magnified benefit from its rich nucleic acids and other healing nutrients.

The liquid extract "has an overall positive effect on the body," says Dr. Steenblock. "Since it is in liquid form, it is quickly absorbed by the body. The CGF liquid can also be very beneficial to conditions of the upper intestinal tract such as an irritated esophagus or stomach ulcers. This is because of the direct soothing and healing effects upon the tissues from the concentration of CGF. The chlorella liquid extract often offers immediate results in such upper intestinal tract problems."

Another important use of the liquid extract is as a topical skin application. Rapid healing of diabetic ulcers and other skin conditions has been frequently observed, when generous amounts of CGF liquid extract were applied.

The recommended dose of chlorella liquid extract is one ounce a day. But people who need to prevent illness or heal troublesome ailments can safely increase their dose. Some medical researchers and patients have reported that by taking four to five ounces a day, they note significantly improved health conditions.

How Soon Will Chlorella Work For You?

Everyone who takes chlorella wants an immediate result. And it is possible to get lucky and experience a remarkable upsurge in your health within days of beginning your chlorella program. But most people need a little more time to feel its full effect. Usually, you will experience a noticeable improvement in your health after three months, but there are those who take chlorella for six months before they sense its benefits.

Certain conditions respond rapidly to chlorella. Constipation and bad breath can often improve within one or two days. And diabetic ulcers heal significantly faster when treated with topical applications of chlorella CGF liquid extract. But many other conditions need more time to mend and heal.

Of course, in order to enjoy the true bounty of chlorella's health-giving ability, you must faithfully take it. Don't make the mistake of enjoying enhanced well-being and vitality and then stopping your chlorella regimen. Testimonials from people who took for granted their new level of health and then stopped taking chlorella make clear that they soon regretted that decision. When their health plummeted, they rushed to resume their daily intake of chlorella, keenly aware of the difference it makes in their overall wellness.

To Sum It All Up...

Here are some basic guidelines for getting the most out of chlorella:

- Select a superior brand, preferably one whose cell wall has been treated with the DYNO-Mill™ method.
- Begin slowly. The usual initial amount is five tablets (1 gram) a day. You can take them at meals, but that is not essential.
- Over the next two week, work your way up to fifteen tablets (3 grams) a day. Some people take five tablets three times a day at meals, but if that is not convenient, you may take them any time. If you prefer to take all fifteen tablets at once, feel free to do so.
- If you sense a health problem looming, increase the amount. You can take 20, 30, or even 45 tablets (4-9 grams) a day while you are combating illness.
- If you have chronic health problems or a family history of serious medical problems, take a higher daily dose. Again, you may take as many as 45 tablets daily if you are facing severe medical challenges.
- Supplement your tablets with chlorella liquid extract, especially if you are over 60 years old or suffering from chronic illness. The usual dose is one ounce daily. To support your individual needs, you may want to take up to four or five ounces daily.
- Give children one tablet for each year of age. For instance, seven-year-olds should get seven tablets. The tablets can be crushed and added to soft foods.
- Be patient. Allow as long as six months to notice a significant upsurge in your health.
- Keep taking your chlorella regimen faithfully. Just as you eat every day to satisfy your body's requirements, so should you take chlorella.
- Drink plenty of water to aid in the detoxifying process.

CHAPTER 26
Superfood for the 21st Century

Chlorella is 2.5 billion years old, yet in some ways, its story is just beginning. Until the late 1970's, chlorella was not allowed in the United States, because its extraordinarily tough cell wall made it difficult to digest. Then came the discovery of the patented DYNO-Mill™ process, which pulverizes the cell wall, hugely increasing digestibility while retaining the integrity of the nutrients inside. A new era of chlorella had begun.

Since then, research in Japan, the United States, Israel and other countries has uncovered massive evidence of chlorella's health-giving powers. Scientists have investigated its impact on virtually every aspect of the body, finding ever more ways that chlorella protects and supports health.

Natural Nourishment for Every Part of Your Body

Here are just a few of the many benefits that chlorella is now known to confer:

- stimulates the immune system, increasing resistance to disease.
- promotes healthy digestion and good bowel health.
- protects the brain from Alzheimer's and memory loss.
- escorts toxins out of the body, including pesticides and heavy metals.
- mends damaged tissue and diabetic ulcers and wounds.
- promotes normal blood pressure levels and good cholesterol health.
- protects against cancer and helps to prevent cancer's recurrence.
- boosts energy levels and increases cellular efficiency.
- reverses the aging process and promotes longevity.

Ten Million People Take Chlorella Every Day

Today, over ten million people around the world take chlorella to improve their health. Chlorella is the largest-selling supplement in Japan, and every year, its popularity continues to soar in the United States.

As clinical data continues to pour in, scientists are realizing that chlorella has a gigantic contribution to make to the human story. Well-suited for growing conditions in space, chlorella may someday be a food staple of planetary voyagers. Here on earth, chlorella may provide a marvelous protein source for underdeveloped countries suffering from food scarcity. And in Western countries plagued with overly-processed food and toxic environments, chlorella can serve as an unmatched source of healthful nutrition, purifying, healing, protecting and revitalizing.

The Road to Health Begins Here

People who take chlorella never want to go without it again. Their ferocious loyalty to their little green tablets springs from the miraculous changes it makes in their lives. Once you too have made the journey from exhaustion to vitality, from anxiety to serenity, from illness to health, you will never, ever, want to go back.

We invite you to begin your journey now.

CHAPTER 27
Chlorella Users
Speak Their Mind

"When I Found Chlorella, It Was My Lucky Day"

"I am so glad that chlorella found me — I don't remember how, but that was my lucky day. I have been taking it for nearly a year and my colon problem has disappeared and my allergy problem is much better. I am 82 years old, but I feel more like 62. I have more energy and I am on the go constantly. Thank you, chlorella!"

—EDITH KERN, LAKE ISABELLA, CALIFORNIA

Back Pain Better

"Within 1½ days of starting chlorella, my hip and back pain decreased tremendously. When taking regular daily amounts, I feel more energetic, with less hip and back pain."

—JAMES NELSON, TACOMA, WASHINGTON

"I Have So Much Energy, I Feel 20 Years Younger"

"There are so many rewarding benefits I have received from using chlorella. I now have full use of my hands. Before I couldn't use a wrench or tie my shoes. I was unable to get around well because my right knee would cave in and bending down on my knee was out of the question. My once prominent varicose veins have now drastically reduced in size. Also, I've noticed that my body odors (all) have almost diminished. I have so much agility now, I can do exercises with little restriction. I have so much energy, I feel 20 years younger!"

—JOHN LELLO, SAN JOSE, CALIFORNIA

No Longer Needs A Cane

"I honestly believe chlorella is helping me. I haven't been able to walk without a cane for over a year. Now I don't need my cane."

—HAZEL MARR, SANTA ROSA, CALIFORNIA

Lower Blood Pressure, Cholesterol…And Weight

"I started taking chlorella in 6/87. It has helped me with weight loss from 175 to 150, maintain blood pressure to near normal, lower cholesterol from 243 to 180."

—JOHN POOLE, DIXON, WYOMING

It's Fantastic!

"Chlorella is fantastic. It builds up my immune system…I almost never catch colds. The high protein content and nutrients keep me from eating unwholesome foods. I regard this whole food with great reverence. I will not stop buying or eating chlorella."

—ROBERT MITCHELL, WOODINVILLE, WASHINGTON

Sleep and Comfort

"Since I have been taking chlorella, I sleep better and I'm regular. I've been sharing with a friend. She is always saying how much better she feels."

—MARIAN MATHEWSON, BELLEVAL, WASHINGTON

It Keeps Him Going Strong

"Last week I was traveling and working approximately 18 hours every day. I believe the energy I received from chlorella is what kept me going without feeling overly tired."

—HAROLD ROSEBRUGH, THOUSAND OAKS, CALIFORNIA

"The Energy Has Been A Blessing"

"I have had a lot of trouble making many trips to the bathroom at night and to my surprise, I slept eight hours for the first time in many years. I have much more energy than I could think possible. My overall health has been much improved…I am sure it is a Godsend."

—ROBERT WALKER, MADISONVILLE, KENTUCKY

Alleviating Stress With Chlorella Extract

"I have been taking the chlorella extract honey flavor before going to work. The energy, calmness and smoothness has been a blessing during the hectic hours of waitressing."

—MARLENE LIED, BOCA RATON, FLORIDA

"I Will Never Stop Taking Chlorella"

"The biggest thing I noticed for me is for the very first time in my life I have nice long and strong fingernails. I'm 45 years old and I have never had nice nails…I will never stop taking chlorella."

—CAROLYN ATWOOD, RENTON, WASHINGTON

Hard At Work and Healthy

"I had an enlarged thyroid and was extremely tired all the time. Walking up stairs left my heart racing and cuts on my hands would not heal by themselves. I seemed to always have the cold or the flu. My first source of chlorophyll was in wheat grass juice. Then I learned chlorella had larger amounts. My thyroid is almost back to normal size. My energy is fantastic. Colds and flu are almost non-existent or very mild. Any cuts heal in record time. I wouldn't have been able to work as hard as I do as a mail carrier these last two years if it were not for chlorella for energy…"

—DEE DEVRIES, HEBRON, ILLINOIS

Miraculous Healing

"I started taking chlorella for energy but soon realized that was not the only benefit. I had a fungus around my thumbnail for several years. After about two weeks, it was gone. I had two warts on my thumb for many years. Now they are gone and the skin is smooth…The healing from this is miraculous."

—SHELBY WOODEN, BRANSON, MISSOURI

Nothing Helped…Until Chlorella

"I had swelling and pain in both feet and legs due to injury (World War II). Nothing has given me any relief. Medication, acupuncture, surgery, physical therapy, nothing helped. Then approximately three months on chlorella there has been less pain. No swelling, some relief, which is all I asked for."

—ADOLFO ARELLANES, SAN FRANCISCO, CALIFORNIA

Younger-Looking, Healthier Skin

"Since I have been taking chlorella, I have more energy than I had in fifteen years (I am 46 now). I had a skin problem since I was in high school and it is clearing up real good. I look much younger."

—CURTIS WILLIAMS, NORWALK, CALIFORNIA

"Instead of Going to the Candy Machine, I Take Chlorella"

"I am called on to work a double shift, 18 hours. Instead of going to the candy machine, I keep chlorella in my lunch bag, take five more and I breeze through the next eight hours. Inside and outside I feel great."

—WILLIAM ALLISON, MANCHESTER, NEW HAMPSHIRE

Vitality and Energy Sky Rocketed

"I was diagnosed with ovarian cancer in 1994. I was constantly developing toxemia from my disease and the effects of it. After six months of taking chlorella, I have suffered no toxemia and my doctor can't believe it. My vitality and energy have sky rocketed and I no longer take estrogen or prescriptions to curtail my symptoms. They're gone."

—PAMELA LANNING, TORRANCE, CALIFORNIA

More Endurance

"Since I began taking chlorella consistently, my bowel movements are very regular and less discomforting. Endurance during physical fitness workouts has improved, helping to stabilize heart rate and blood pressure. I have tried quite a few natural herbal products by chlorella is by far the best yet."

—ERNEST OSBORNE, LAPUENTE, CALIFORNIA

Rash is Gone

"For years I had a tiny little rash on my shoulders and upper arms. After a few weeks on the tablets, it disappeared and has not returned. My appetite has decreased and that is certainly welcome because I have always had to be careful of my eating."

—CAROL CUTHILL, FAYETTERVILLE, NORTH CAROLINA

"Cured A Viral Infection I Never Got Over"

"Last year I had a viral infection that I never seemed to get over. For months afterwards I was so tired that I was actually taking naps each day at lunch so that I could finish my days work. Had all the blood tests - no apparent problems. Then out of desperation, I tried chlorella and almost immediately had new found energy again. Now I have energy to exercise at lunch again. Thanks chlorella!"

—JACKIE CUMMINGS, WALLA WALLA, WASHINGTON

Energy and a Sense of Well-Being

"I took chlorella tablets which were offered by my friend, and noticed in a very short while that I experienced a greater sense of well-being and energy. I would recommend them to anyone who wants to feel better."

—RANDALL WINTON, LOS ANGELES, CALIFORNIA

Looking Good at 91

"Yesterday morning I walked into church and was greeted with "What have you been doing with yourself? You look wonderful! Keep it up whatever it is!"…I replied to these questions by saying "Chlorella is the answer."…You may also be interested to know that my 91st birthday was just celebrated and I am looking forward to many more happy birthdays."

—MILDRED CLARK, ROCK ISLAND, ILLINOIS

Helps With Diabetes

"I am 71 years old and have diabetes. I have days when glucose readings are high. I found out if I take ten chlorella tablets that within a half hour, I am energetic again and ready to go."

—PATSY DAVIDSON, BEAVERTON, OREGON

"My Energy Level Has Really Increased"

"After taking chlorella for over two years, I can honestly say that I feel more fit and healthy than ever before in my life. As a full-time professional fishing guide, I spend over 275 days a year in the water. My energy level has really increased…I also lift weights, power walk and play tournament caliber table tennis on a weekly basis. Being over 50 doesn't mean you can't improve your quality of life and fitness. Chlorella is an invaluable asset for my health."

—ALLEN CHRISTENSON, AUSTIN, TEXAS

Deep Cut Healed Without Stitches

"I am employed in the construction field and got a deep cut with a piece of light weight galvanized metal. I knew that this cut should require three to four stitches, having received stitches before. At that time, I was taking 10 chlorella tablets daily. I increased the dosage to 15 and in a matter of four days saw a remarkable healing rate with only the aid of a bandaid and no stitches."

—LAREN MADISON, SIMI VALLEY, CALIFORNIA

Feeling Good

"I have been using chlorella for over a year now. I notice that I have infinite energy, kept my slim figure, no illnesses in this time, great overall sense of well-being."

—ARIANNE KOREN, CATHEDRAL CITY, CALIFORNIA

Allergies Are Gone

"I'm writing to say I'm feeling better than I've ever felt. I had osteoporosis, arthritis, allergies, gout and H.B.P. I've had pain in my whole body. I could hardly get up and walk. But since I started taking chlorella, I was able in a few weeks to notice the difference...I sleep better. Walk better. Hardly any pains. I'm more energetic. Think better. Allergies are gone...It's a miracle...I can't say enough about chlorella. It's solved my problems."

—RUTH BOROWSKI, MEDINA, OHIO

"I am 70 Years Old and Energetic"

"I am 70 years old and energetic. I credit this to taking chlorella. Previously, I had trouble having the energy to do all that is for one to do, plus work four hours a day, and being able to stay awake after dinner."

—ANGELA MILLER, LOS ANGELES, CALIFORNIA

Breathing With Ease

"I have suffered from a bronchial problem all my life. Since using chlorella, I do not cough as much, also the mucus and congestion I suffered from has been reduced to almost nothing. It is such a pleasure to breathe with such ease."

—ROBERT HURLEY, LOS ANGELES, CALIFORNIA

Relief From Fatigue

"I had chronic fatigue when I started taking chlorella. Yes, I can feel the difference. When I don't take it, I'm literally exhausted, but if I keep taking it, I feel pretty good.."

—BARBARA CONKLIN, CHESAPEAKE BEACH, MARYLAND

Feeling Balanced and Strong

"After taking chlorella, I find my health in stronger physical and mental form, and my mood to be more stable on "those days" women tend to be dragon ladies because of the hormone imbalance. My energy level is higher and I feel more alert. Overall, chlorella is an excellent balancer and cleanser for the body and mind."

—LORRAINE ANDRADE, MONTEBELLO, CALIFORNIA

Old Symptoms Returned When She Stopped Taking Chlorella

"I stopped taking chlorella for a month and all my old symptoms returned. Hair falling out, vertigo, breaking nails, eyesight, aging skin, colon got worse and got the sniffles."

—DOROTHY ALDERSON, DANIA, FLORIDA

Peace of Mind and Clarity

"My position in property management does create stress. I have noticed that when I have the chlorella regularly, I have a clear head, more alert, but never hyper. This is the honest to God truth."

—LOU ARRBOLA, LOS ANGELES, CALIFORNIA

A Teenager Now Can Focus In School

"My Mom and I both take chlorella daily. She's concerned about my nutritional needs as a teenager. I've been taking chlorella for over a year now. I've grown four inches this year. I used to have a problem with concentration during class. I'm working on track, my grades have improved and I have fewer sick days. I feel chlorella has made a big difference."

—JARED ALDRICH, CANYON, CALIFORNIA

Sinus Headaches Gone

"For years I have battled with sinus headaches daily. I tried everything with no success. Finally spirulina seemed to help, but only temporarily. Then I tried chlorella. Not only did my energy level pick up, but my sinus headaches were gone, leaving me free of daily doses of Advil and nausea that accompanied the headaches."

—GRACE BUKOWSKI, VALINDA, CALIFORNIA

Cured Sweat Problem

"Harvey had changed deodorant and tried everything and still he would sweat and wet a shirt on the right side. Since taking chlorella, the shirt is now dry. That is so wonderful."

—DELORES AND HARVEY BASS, SHAWNEE, OKLAHOMA

Pain Lifted and Can Smile Again

"I just wanted to write and let you know about my results in taking chlorella for the past 3½ months. I have rheumatism, osteoporosis, and fibromyalgia and have experienced a lot of intense, constant pain for the last five years. After using your chlorella, my pain has let up to where I can smile again."

—GRACE BERMUDES, LATAH, WASHINGTON

Improved Hearing and Eyesight

"I can't say enough in such little space about the tremendous turn-around in my health after starting on chlorella. My hearing, my eyesight, my inactive lifestyle; in fact, every part of my body feels like it's being cleansed. I could write a book about chlorella. It's increased my level of energy, alertness, improved my memory, etc. I am 76 years old and feel like I am 38 again…I love it."

—LUCILLE BOLD, SACRAMENTO, CALIFORNIA

It's a Silent Worker

"It's a silent worker. Seems as though it's not doing much good, but just go without it and you see the difference. I am 92 years old, I've gone without the chlorella for a while and I was sorry I did. Won't do it again."

—FRANCES HELLMAN, COLBERT, GEORGIA

Scalp Condition Cured

"Over a period of six years, and at a cost of several thousand dollars, I have been treated for bumps in my head by three dermatologists in three states. They each prescribed a medicated shampoo, which treated the symptom, but never the cause. After taking 15 tablets per day of chlorella for a period of three months, the bumps disappeared."

—LEROY GAILLARD, BIRMINGHAM, ALABAMA

Relief from Irritable Bowel Syndrome

"I have irritable bowel syndrome and chlorella has made such a difference that I do want to ever be without it. My elimination is so much better. I am not constipated as much and my energy went up because of it."

—CHRISTINE GORDAN, SAN DIEGO, CALIFORNIA

No Joint Pain

"Since my chiropractor prescribed chlorella and other nutritional supplements, I have had no joint pain, fewer leg cramps, and I have been healed of my sciatic pinched nerves and my deteriorating discs have improved, too."

—CHIYETO OKAMOTO, LOS ANGELES, CALIFORNIA

Pet Owners Praise Chlorella

No More Hot Spots!

"Before using chlorella, my 9-year-old dog was plagued with hot spots, and ear infections. After 2 weeks of using chlorella, she cleared up and acted vibrant."

—KATHY KNIGHT, PANAMA CITY, FLORIDA

No Longer Picking at Her Fur!

"Earlier this past spring, my cat Abbie started pulling out her fur by big globs. Then she would lick the bare spots raw. I started her on (chlorella) and she soon stopped pulling her fur out and the new fur came in soft and shiny. Abbie is allergic to fleas and she doesn't even scratch anymore."

—EVELYN RAMOS, SAN JOSE, CALIFORNIA

Immune System Back on Track!

"Smokey, my 12-year-old dog, became infected with Demodectic. After about 5 weeks of chlorella, Smokey was making a speedy recovery, and the hair started to grow back."

—SHARON KAPTEINA, AURORA, ILLINOIS

Plays Like a Puppy at 10 Years Old!

"I started my collie on chlorella because of an itching, and thinning coat. Now, while she is on her second box of (wafers), her eyes are bright, and she plays like a puppy. You would never know she is 10 years old."

—Ione Swope, Coral Gables, Florida

Energetic and Healthy at 11!

"My dog Jasper was ailing from hot spots and allergies. She takes a pet chlorella tablet in the morning and the evening. She started on them five years ago. She is now 11 years old, energetic and in great health! She looks forward to (chlorella wafers) as treats every day."

—Lisa Birkenberger, Cedar Rapids, Iowa

Need for Greens...Satisfied

"If I don't give my cats their chlorella, they eat my plants...When I have left the chlorella out, they have torn the package open to get to the chlorella."

—Sandra Bostwick, Portland, Oregon

Appendix 1: References

1. A Chlorella Experiment with Maritime Self-Defense Forces Members, **Scientific Reports on Chlorella in Japan**, 1992, Silpaque Publishing, Inc. , Kyoto, Japan.

2. Enhanced Resistance Against Eschericia Coli Infection by Subcutaneous Administration of Hot Water Extract of Chlorella Vulgaris in Cyclophosphamide-Treated Mice, **Cancer Immunology Immunotherapy**, 1990, 32: pp. 1-7.

3. Effect of Chlorella Vulgaris Extracts on Murine Cytomegalovirus, **Nat Immun Cell Growth Regul.**, 1990, 9: pp. 121-128

4. Hot Water Extracts of Chlorella Vulgaris Reduce Opportunistic Infection With Listeria Monocytogenes in C57BL/6 Mice Infected with LP-BM5 Murine Leukemia Viruses, **Int. Journal Immunopharmacology (England)**, June 1995, 17(6): pp. 505-512

5. Dietary Chlorella Pyrenoidosa for Patients with Malignant Glioma: Effects of Immuno-competence, Quality of Life, and Survival, **Phytotherapy Research**, 1990, 4 (6): pp. 220-231

6. Protective effect of an acidic glycoprotein obtained from culture of chlorella vulgaris against myelosuppression by 5-fluorouracil, **Cancer Immunology, Immonotherapy**, June 1996, 42: pp. 268-271.

7. **Chlorella, Natural Medicinal Algae** by Dr. David Steenblock, p. 20 referencing 'Effect of chlorella on fecal and urinary excretion in "Itai-Itai",' **Japan Jrnl of Hyg.**, 1975, 30 (1): pp. 77

8. Absorption and excretion of cadmium by the rat administered cadmium-containing chlorella, **Eisei Kagaku**, 1978, 24: pp. 7182-7186

9. Effect of Zinc Administration on cadmium-induced suppression of natural killer cell activity in mice, **Canada Immunology Letters**, 1989, 22(4): pp. 287-291

10. Results of Dental amalgam removal and mercury detoxification using DMPS and neural therapy, **Alternative Therapies in Health & Medicine**, July 2000, 6(4): pp 49-55

11. Alternative Medicine Digest, May 1994.

12. Mercury removed by immobilized algae in batch culture systems, **J. Appl. Physical**, 1990, 2(23): pp. 223-230.

13. Consumer's Union, publisher of Consumer Reports, Feb. 1999. Based on USDA pesticide data program (PDP) 1994-1997

14. Detoxification of chlordecone poisoned rats with chlorella and chlorella derived sporopollenin, **Drug and Chemical Toxicology**, 1984, 7(1): pp. 57-71

15. Chlorella Accelerates Dioxin Excretion in Rats, **Am. Soc for Nutritional Sciences**, Sept. 1999, 129 (9): pp 1731-6

16. **Chlorella, Natural Medicinal Algae** by Dr. David Steenblock, Page 20.

17. Inhibition of 2-amino-3-methylimidazo [4,5-f]quinoline (IQ)—DNA binding in rats given chlorophyllin: dose—response and time-course studies in the liver and colon, **Carcinogenesis**, 1994, 15(4), pp. 763-766.

18. It's Not Easy Being Green: Chlorophyll Being Tested, **Jnl of the National Cancer Inst.**, 1995.

19. Dietary Chlorophyllin is a potent inhibitor of aflatoxin B1 hepatocarcinogenesis in rainbow trout, **Cancer Research**, 1992, 55(1): pp. 57-62

20. Protection by Chlorophyllin and indole-3-carbinol against 2-amino-1-methyl-6-phenylimidazo[4,5-b] pyridine (PhIP)-induced DNA adducts and colonic aberrant crypts in the F344 rat, **Carcinogenesis**, 1995, 16: pp. 2931-2937.

21. Inhibitory Effects of Chlorophyllin on Chemically Induced Mutagenesis and Carcinogenisis, **Ann N Y Acad Sci (United States)**, Sept. 1995, 768: pp. 246-249.

22. Novel glycoprotein obtained from Chlorella vulgaris strain CK22 shows anitmetastatic immunopoteniation, **Cancer Immunol. Immunother**, 1998, 45: pp. 313-320.

23. A Water-Soluble antitumor glycoprotein from Chlorella Vulgaris, **Planta Medica**, 1996, 62: pp. 423-426.

24. The Effects of Chlorella Vulgaris in the protection of mice infected with Listeria monocytogenes, role of natural killer cells, **Immunopharmacology and Immunotoxicology**, 1999, 21(3) 609-619

25. Effects of long-term administration of chlorella preparations on the advancement of aging in humans and laboratory animals, **Scientific Reports on Chlorella in Japan**, 1992. Silpaque publishing, Inc. Kyoto, Japan

26. Chlorella Natural Medicinal Algae, Page 22 referencing: Use of chlorophyllin in the care of geriatric patients. **J am Geriatrics Soc**, 1980, 28: pp. 46-47, Deodorization of colostomies with chlorophyllin, **Rev. Gastroentorol.**, 1951,18: p. 602.

27. **Chlorella, Gem of the Orient** by Dr. Bernard Jensen, p. 26

28. Chlorophyll use in tissue culture, **Jrnl of Lab and Clinical Med**, 1944, 29: pp. 241-246

29. **Chlorella, Natural Medicinal Algae** by Dr. David Steenblock, p. 15, referencing Smith & Livingston, Wound Healing, **Am J Surg**, 1945, 67: pp. 30-39

30. **Chlorella Jewel of the Far East** by Dr. Bernard Jensen, p.80 referencing The treatment of peptic ulcer by chlorella, **Nihon Iji Shimpo**, 1962.

31. Experience in using chlorella in treating refractory wounds, **Medical Consultation and New Remedies**, 1966.

32. Effect of long-term administration of chlorella tablets on hyperlipidemia, **Jrnl of Japanese Soc. of Nutr. and Food Science**, 1990; 43(3): pp. 167-173

33. Dietary Supplementation with chlorella pyrenoidosa produces positive results in patients with cancer or suffering from certain common chronic illnesses, **Townsend Letter for Doctors & Patients**, 2001; 211-212: pp.74-80

34. Title: Effect of Dried, Powdered Chlorella Vulgaris on Experimental Atherosclerosis and Alimentary Hypercholesterolemia in Cholesterol fed Rabbits, **Artery**, 1987, 14(2): pp. 76-84

35. **Chlorella, Natural Medicinal Algae** by Dr. David Steenblock, Page 32 references: "Effect of chlorella on human pulse wave velocity," 1985, conducted by Kanazawa Medical University, Dept of Serology.

36. Detection and control of high blood pressure in the community: Do we need a wake-up call?, **Hypertension**, Sep 1999, 34(3): pp. 466-71

37. Effects of chlorella alkali extract on blood pressure in SHR, **Artery**, 1978, 19 (4): pp. 622-623

38. **Chlorella, Natural Medicinal Algae** by Dr. David Steenblock, p. 20

39. Brain thiamine, its phosphate esters and its metabolizing enzymes in Alzheimer's

References

disease, **Ann Neurol.**, 1996, 39: pp 585-91

40. **The Brain Wellness** Plan by Lombard & Germano, p. 78

41. **Chlorella, Natural Medicinal Algae** by Dr. David Steenblock, p. 21 referencing "The quality of the protein of unicellular green algae and their effect in preventing liver necrosis," **Physiol Chem**, 1956, 305: pp. 182-191

42. Effect of chlorella on the levels of glycogen triglyceride and cholesterol in ethionine treated rats, **J. Formosan Med Assoc.**, 1980, 78: pp. 1-10

43. Oral administration of hot water extracts of chlorella vulgaris reduces IgE production against milk casein in mice, **Int. Jrnl. of Immunopharmacology**, 1999, 21: pp. 311-323

44. Clinical effect of chlorella vulgaris E-25 on young children with atopic dermatitis, **Pasken Journal**, 1997, 9-10: pp. 11-14

45. Evaluation of Radioprotective Action of a Mutant (E-25) Form of Chlorella Vulgaris in Mice, **Japan Radiation Research Society**, 1993, 34: pp.277-284

46. Post-exposure radioprotection by Chlorella vulgaris (E-25) in mice, **Indian Journal of Experimental Biology**, Aug. 1995, 33: pp. 612-615

47. Immunomodulation by Unicellular Green Algae (Chlorella Pyrenoidosa) in Tumor Bearing Mice, **Journal of Ethnopharmacology**, 1988, 24: pp. 135-146

48. Oral Administration of Chlorella Vulgaris Augments Concomitant Anti-Tumor Immunity **Immunopharmacology and Immunotoxicology**, 1990, 12 (2), pp. 277-291

49. Chlorophyll in treatment of ulcers, **Syphilol**, 1943, 49: pp. 849-851

50. Chlorophyll: An experimental study of its water soluble derivatives in wound healing, **Amer. J. Surg**, 1943, 67 pp. 30-39

51. Nutritional treatment program and age-related macular degeneration: improved vision one year later, **Townsend Letter**, 1997, 162: pp. 80-81

52. Chlorophyllin as an effective antioxidant against membrane damage in vitro and ex vivo, **Biochimica et Biophysica Acta (Netherlands)**, Sept 27 2000, 1487 (2-3): pp. 113-27

53. The relation between antioxidants and memory performance in the old and very old, **Jrnl. of the Amer. Ger. Soc.**, June 1997, 45(6): pp. 718-724

54. Augmentation of Host Defense by a Unicellular Green Alga, Chlorella Vulgaris, to Escherichia Coli Infection, **Infection and Immunity**, 1986, 53 (2): pp. 267-271

55. Chlorella vulgaris culture supernatant (CVS) reduces psychological stress-induced apoptosis in thymocytes of mice, **Intl. Jrnl. of Immunopharmacology (England)**, Nov 2000, 22(11): pp.877-85

56. **Chlorella Gem of the Orient** by Dr. Bernard Jensen, p. 143

Index

Abel, Jr., Robert, Dr., 91-92
acidophilus, 38
aflatoxin, 24, 105
aging, 33-36
  free radicals, 33-36, 50-51, 93-95
  nucleic acids, 10, 34
  nutrition, 33-36, 97-99
alcohol, 12, 61-62, 87
allergies, 65-67
  aid to pets, 105, 123-124
  testimonials, 115, 120, 123, 124
aluminum, 16, 50, 84
Alzheimer's, 49-51
  chlorella study, 35, 49
  free radicals, 12, 50
  toxins, 16, 18, 19
American diet:
  problems with, 11, 21, 22, 23, 30, 37, 45, 46, 98, 102,
American Heart Association, 45, 48
American Institute of Nutrition, 10
American Journal of Surgery, 41
amino acids, 28, 29, 91
Annals of Neurology, 50
antibiotics, 41-43, 88
antioxidants, 12, 28, 29, 50, 91, 92, 93-95
arginine, 29
arteries, hardening of, 46-48, 87, 93
asthma, 65-67, 101
autoimmunity, 65
bacterial infection, 8, 25, 41-43, 70, 80, 88
Beijerinck, M.W., 4
beta-carotene content in chlorella, 29
  function of, 29, 94
body odors, 39
  testimonials, 115, 122
bone marrow colony forming units, 9, 69, 71
bowel, 37-39, 62, 79-81
  testimonials, 118, 123
brain and memory, 35, 93-96
  Alzheimer's, 49-51, 84
  tumors, 9, 72-73
Brain Wellness Plan, 49, 51, 77, 95
brand selection, 107-109
cadmium, 16-18, 84
  in cigarette smoke, 47-48
cancer, 69-73
  carcinogens, 21-24
  chlorella as adjunct to treatment, 9, 69-73
  effect of environmental toxins, 15-17
  tumor-related studies, 9, 24, 71-73
Cancer Immunology& Immunotherapy, 8
Cancer Research Journal, 24

candidiasis, 18, 78
Carcinogenesis, 24
carotenes/carotenoids, 29, 91
cell wall (chlorella):
  detoxification, 11-12, 16, 38, 66, 83-85
  digestibility problems, 4, 107
  processing, 4-5, 107-108
cellular energy, 93-94
chemical sensitivities, 65-67, 83-85
chemotherapy, 9, 69-70, 72-73
children:
  growth enhancement, 101
  special health concerns, 19, 21, 53, 55, 66-67, 75, 80, 101-103
  usage of chlorella, 67, 102-103
chlordecone, 23, 85
chlorella growth factor (chlorella extract):
  Definition and usage, 4, 27-28, 42-43, 62, 69-73, 88-89, 102, 109-111
  Studies Using, 8-9, 18, 24-25, 42, 47, 49, 58, 66, 69-73, 80, 95
Chlorella, Gem of the Orient (Jensen), 1,28
Chlorella, Jewel of the Far East (Jensen), 62
Chlorella, Natural Medicinal Algae
(Steenblock), 16, 18, 35, 46, 55, 85, 107
chlorophyll:
  as a detoxifier, 16, 19, 23-24, 28
  as an antibiotic, 42
  as an antioxidant, 94
  content in chlorella, 3-4, 28, 31
  control of constipation, 38-39, 79
  use in odor control, 39
  use for sinitis, 54-55
  use in tissue repair, 28, 41-43, 87-89
chlorophyllin, 24, 39
cholesterol, 45-48, 62, 93
  testimonial, 116
chronic fatigue syndrome, 15, 18, 19, 77-78,
  testimonial, 120
cigarette smoke, 12, 17, 47-48, 84
cirrhosis of the liver, 61, 62
Clofibrate, 46, 93
colon, 23, 38, 79-80
  testimonials 115, 121
common cold, 53-55, 72, 102, 109
  testimonials, 99, 116, 117
constipation, 37-39, 79-80, 83, 110
  testimonials, 116, 118, 123
cravings, 3, 30, 118
Crohn's disease, 79-81
Cyclophosphamide, 69-70
cytomegalovirus, 8, 70
DDT, 16, 21-22

MacArthur Foundation, 33
macular degeneration, 91-92
magnesium, 29, 91, 92
malnutrition, 10-11, 33-34, 97-98
Mayo Clinic, 80, 87
Mayo Clinic Family Health Book, 7
meat as a source of toxins, 23-25, 30, 80, 83
Medical College of Virginia, 2-3, 9, 13, 54, 58, 72-73
medication interactions, 42, 69-73, 88, 105
memory loss, 35, 49-51, 83, 84, 93-96
Merchant, Randall E., Dr., 2-3, 13, 58, 79, 80
mercury, 16, 17-18, 50, 83-84
methionine, 91
mitochondria, 93-94
Miyazaki Medical College, 8
NASA, 29
natural killer cells, 8, 25
neurotoxins, 15-19, 21-22, 83-85
New York Times, 21, 22
normalizing action of chlorella, 2-3
nucleic acids:
  content in chlorella, 10, 28, 34
  functions, 10, 34, 62
nutrients in chlorella, 3-4, 27-29
pain: causes of, 17, 18, 42, 57-59, 65, 75, 77-78, 80, 87-88
  testimonials, 34-35, 36, 58-59, 115, 117, 120, 122, 123
pancreas, 61
Patterson, Claire, Ph.D., 15
PCBs, 16, 18, 23, 107
pesticide use, 15, 21-22
  detoxification of, 16, 22-23, 84-85, 107
pet chlorella, 105-106
  testimonials, 123-124
physical properties of chlorella, 3-4
Pore, Dr., 23, 85
pregnancy: benefits of chlorella, 18-19, 25, 102,
production of chlorella, 4-5
protein:
  content in chlorella, 4, 11, 28-29, 108
  deficiency in, 10-11, 29-30
  function of, 28-29, 79
pyorhhea, 41
radiation treatments, 71-73
rashes, 65-67
  testimonial, 35, 118
respiratory problems, 9, 15, 53-55, 65-67, 72
  testimonials, 35, 120
Ridpath & Davis, Drs., 54
Rockefeller Foundation, 4
Rooke, Thomas W., Dr., 87

Rosenbaum, Micheal E., Dr., 16, 29, 103
seafood as a source of toxins, 17-18, 25, 65, 83
silver amalgam fillings, 15, 18, 19, 83-84
sinus condition, 54-55, 65-67
  testimonial, 121
sleep problems, 57-59, 70, 75-76
  testimonials, 116, 120
spirulina: comparison to chlorella, 4, 11, 16, 31
Steenblock, David, Dr., 35, 46, 106, 107, 109, 110
  on CGF and healing of ulcers, 42-43, 88-89
  on detoxification, 16-19, 85
  on Epstein-Barr infection, 75-76
  recipe for sinus condition, 55
stomach, 41-43, 88-89, 110
stress, 58, 95-96
  testimonials, 116, 121
Successful Aging, 33-34
suggestions on chlorella use, 109-111
superoxide dismutase (SOD), 94-95
taurine, 91
T-cells, 8, 10, 24, 29, 72
The American Cancer Society, 24
tissue repair:
  diabetic ulcers, 87-88
  wounds, 41-43, 62, 79
Townsend Letter for Doctors and Patients, 92
Triglycerides, 45
tumor growth, 24, 71-72
ulcerative colitis, 79-81
ulcers, 41-43, 87-89
uranium, 18
viral infections, 8, 53-55, 63, 70, 75-76, 109
vision problems, 91-92
  testimonials, 121, 122
vitamin A, 12, 29, 91
vitamin B-1 (thiamine), 29, 50
vitamin B-12, 29, 50, 80, 97, 98
vitamin B-2 (riboflavin), 50
vitamin B-6 (pyridoxine), 11, 29, 50, 77, 97, 98
vitamin E, 29, 97, 98
vitamin B-group, 38, 50, 91
weight gain: sustaining healthy level, 3, 17, 101, 107
weight loss, 2-3, 30
  testimonials, 95, 116, 118
Weingarten & Payson, Drs., 39
white blood cell deficiency, 7-10, 69-73
wound healing, 41-43, 62, 79, 87-89
  testimonials, 117, 119
Young & Beregi, Drs., 39
zinc, 10-11, 17, 29, 51, 77, 91, 92, 97, 98